FOLLOW YOUR BLISS

A Guide to a Powerful Mindset

GREG DYER

ISBN #: 978-1542445368

For permission requests, email Greg Dyer at
Greg@ConsciousGreg.Com or write to the address below:

Greg Dyer Inc.
1961 S Havana St.
Aurora, Co. 80014

www.ConsciousGreg.com

This book is not intended to be a substitute for the medical advice
of a licensed physician. The reader should consult with their
doctor in any matters relating to his/her health.

ೲ Praise for Greg ಛ

"Greg Dyer has an approach to life and writing that comes from a place of heart, powerful intention and love. He is willing to look beyond the surface and dive in to the realms of the spirit to be guided and to guide others that he has the beautiful ability to affect. His intuition and light energy place him in a category of healer and teacher and I feel confident the messages in his writing will positively impact many minds, bodies and spirits for decades to come."

Paula Robbins

Three years ago, after getting a go ahead from my doctor that my degenerative disc was getting better, I was told I could once again get back into the gym.

I was very apprehensive. I walked into Colorado Pro Gym and asked the owner if he could recommend a personal trainer for me. He got in touch with Greg Dyer and told him my health situation. Upon meeting Greg and finding out that he had once battled the same ailment, I was immediately relieved.

I was touting almost a size 35 waist and was about 20 lbs. over my normal weight. I also had a very high BMI.

After working with Greg for those 3 years I am finally where I want to be. I not only made a good friend, but my respect for him as a personal trainer proved to be without a doubt deserving. My quality of life is better because of him. It's not every 67-year-old man who can now do a 5+ minute plank. Thank you Greg!

Len

I've known Greg for about 6 years. We initially became acquainted as I was mid-way in my Weight Watchers program and I wanted to pursue some weight training with the intention of turning some excess flab into muscle and at my age, then 56, I knew it would take a concentrated effort to gain some body 'definition'. With Greg's guidance, I was able to achieve these goals. Greg was able to coax my 'non-confident' mindset into a new persona of confidence about my weight loss success and new appearance. He offered numerous tips on food choices and exercise routines that I carry with me to this day.

Since Greg and I had kept in contact, I was aware of some new directions he was pursuing outside of the typical 'trainer' mode and in January of this year, I asked if he would be interested in being my 'guide' as I wanted to get an 'internal FIX' on my eating disorders and to 'reset' a few parameters going forward. While we both weren't sure how this would work, he agreed to become my 'life coach' in finding a solution and offered his guidance. Again, after 5 months of semi-weekly discussions and confabs, I'm seeing the benefit of our talks as we journey forward together to GOOD HEALTH. Greg not only possesses a vast amount of exercise know-how, but also an incredible new-age theory about your body being in tune with your mind throughout the day, every day! He has showed me that to 'change', I have to step out of my comfort zone and just GO FOR IT...............guilt-free! Sounds crazy, but IT WORKS!

THANKS, my friend, Greg!

JJ

"Thank you Greg Dyer for creating such an inspirational book that has the ability to motivate and help many!"

Robert Raymond
Best Selling Author

Thank you to my contributors

Greg Justice, MA Owner, AYC Health & Fitness Co-founder & CEO, National Corporate Fitness Institute Co-founder & CEO, Scriptor Publishing Group Author, Treadside Manner - Confessions of a Serial Personal Trainer

Robert Raymond, Business Coach & Mentor Achieve Systems

Shari Mitteco, Business Coach & Accountability Partner

Dr. Steve Peisner, Naturopath, Psychologist, Conscious. Body. Movement. Radio Co-Host

Merlijn Wolsink, Body Worker, Conscious. Body. Movement. Radio Co-Host & Co-Creator

Nicole Taryn, Writer, Body Worker, Conscious. Body. Movement. Co-Creator

I'd also like to thank the following:

Roger & Carryn Dyer

Without your support, I don't know if I would get here! Thank you for being my parents, and my friends!

Kathy Basel, Natural Health Expert/ Creator of The Vitality Code

Your constant inspiration and the space you provide really gave me the strength to finish this book! How lucky do you want to get?

Matt Rauzi, CSCS, Gym Owner Colorado's Pro Gym

Without your help and support, I would not have had this great gym and lab in which to see all of this transpiring in my clients, and the rest of the members of Colorado's Pro Gym!

Vanessa Dyer

Thank you for pushing me to do this. I know you may not see what you did this way, but I do.

Thank you to all of my clients. You have all taught me, and continue to teach me so much!

For Aleksa Always!

Follow your Bliss - Greg Dyer

CONTENTS

Follow your Bliss - Greg Dyer

FOLLOW YOUR BLISS FOREWORD

Greg Justice, MA
National Fitness Hall of Fame Inductee

Eckhart Tolle once said, "In today's rush, we all think too much – seek to much – want too much – and forget about the joy of just being."

Follow Your Bliss is about embodiment and "the joy of just being".

Right off the bat, Greg's quote, "If we act authentically who we are, that is what we get back from the universe" caught my attention and set the tone for the book.

As I read Follow Your Bliss, it felt like I was reading Greg's personal journal of growth and development. It was almost as if he was discovering what he calls "Bliss in Embodiment" right before my eyes.

I enjoyed Greg's approach, with his collection of questions and awareness exercises. No matter what's going on in your life, these exercises can help you better understand and navigate throughout your individual journey.

In chapter one, he talks about consciousness as a path to self-awareness. "Be you. Honor you. Love you!"

At the beginning of chapter two, he asks the question, "What would it take to feel proud, confident, and super sexy, not to mention light, easy, and fun in and with your body now?", then gives you helpful suggestions to overcome self-judgment and criticism.

Chapter three is about Movement and Exercise and talks about the importance of enjoying this process. He asks the question, "If it isn't fun, then why are you doing it?"

Next, in chapter four, Greg gives you practical solutions for "Putting all of this into action", as it relates to nutrition, exercise and relationships.

Chapter five brings it all together with one of my all time favorite quotes by Mahatma Gandhi, "Be the change you wish to see in the world." I'm a Christian, and Gandhi practiced Hinduism, but this quote is relevant to all faiths. We don't have control of what other people say or do, but we do have control of how we react. If we practice Gandhi's quote, we take control of our lives by being authentic and start to see others around us change too. "Be the change" is empowering, "be the change" is authentic, "be the change" can change your life... and change the world.

Read *Follow Your Bliss* book with an open heart and an open mind. Greg shares his life lessons throughout this book and gives practical solutions and recommendations...it's up to you to implement them into your life.

Preface

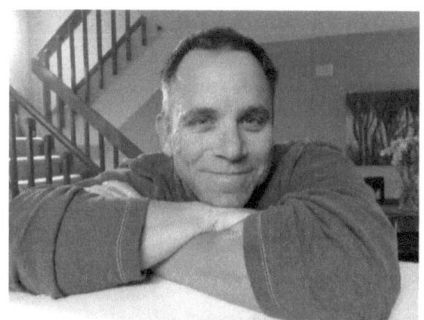

How did I get here
(that is, to the point of writing this all down into a book)?

I have been a personal trainer by trade now for 12-plus years. It's been good: I admit to having a lot of fun, facing some struggle, and enjoying an all-around interesting journey during this part of my life. When I started training people, I was with the woman of my dreams. We had just bought our first house together, just starting to settle into domestic bliss, then...

Boom! I got fired!

I was fired from the company for which I had worked for 8 years.

What to do now?

The aforementioned woman of my dreams said to me, "Go get certified to be a personal trainer. You are good at it!" Then, 3 or so months later, and certification in hand, I set up shop in the local gym and began training people for a living.

I married the woman of my dreams about a year later, and we made some plans to move forward with a family. Our daughter was born about 2 years later, and at that point, most everything felt right with the world. A few cracks in the armor of wedded bliss, but no more than I'd ever heard about from others' experiences. We struggle with money.

Yeah, I know — who doesn't? Of course, financial woes can break up a relationship. I know this. I read about it all the time. But we will be fine. We will work it out. Big dreams are hatched between us.

Besides, all along, something else was happening.

See, I had married a great woman, but she had expectations — expectations of me, of herself, and of others around her. If those expectations weren't met, she struggled with that. She would push people out. In fact, she pushed me out, over and over again. These were dark moments in my life, but these details are important to the story here. Those moments taught me more than I ever realized about expectations, projections, and judgments, and how these are disruptors to bliss.

Ultimately, it wasn't the expectation that someone had on me, but rather the expectations I put on myself to meet the expectations of another. And we're talking about situations where in order to meet those expectations, I would be required to act in a way that was different from my true self. I would have to handle situations like someone else might, rather than how I normally would. It's like cutting parts of yourself off to fit into a car: you may want to ride in that car, but to squeeze into it will mean hiding or even getting rid of parts of your true self.

This can never really work out. Not if you're looking for bliss in this experience! It can't work for you, and it can't work for the people with whom you have relationships. This is what happened to me. I have described the sequence of events that caused the split behind these dark moments in my life.

The separation came first, then of course a divorce. The separation hurt, then the divorce was just closing the door on that part of my life about a year later. I thought she had done this, that this was because of choices she had made. No matter how I looked at it, my world was shattered. Here I was, living in my gracious friend's spare bedroom, sharing it every other day with my 5-year old daughter (thankfully she remains a constant in my life), and wondering what had just happened?

There were plenty of times when I thought of suicide. Plenty of times — like every day.

I wanted out of this. I even asked God to take me out, to remove me from this alternate timeline. I started drinking more, I stopped working out, and I looked for things to do to just numb out and escape what was happening.

I had tools at my disposal at the time for digging out, but I chose not to see them, and I chose not to use them. I had been through a few Access Consciousness classes, and knew that asking questions was how I would find my way through this[1].

I also had a few friends who did stick around, and they asked questions for me, just to make sure that I was okay. (If you are reading this, you know who you are. And you are wonderful. Thank you!)

When I did start asking questions again, it was from a place of anger. But that is okay, too. Anger is one of the interesting feelings we get to experience here. It isn't something to run from, to push down inside, or to hide out of reach. Use the anger. You never know where it may lead you. For me, it led to a single question, asked from that place of anger.

"What else is F---in' possible?"

Usually I asked it with my teeth tightly clenched. Of course, I added the expletive, but...

It began to work! I started seeing things beyond what was happening in the moment.

This one question opened me up to the possibilities in life that existed all around me, all of the time. It was entirely my choice to see them, or not, and to act upon them or not.

The next question was: "How does it get any better than this?"

This popped more open for me. I began collaborating with a friend on the other side of the world on something that eventually became Conscious. Body. Movement, and then resulted in this book! Soon there was an explosion of sticky notes on my wall, all boasting questions. As the questions came to me, I wrote about them, marking down all of the fresh awareness that was emerging in regards to the inquiries. Mind you, I didn't make anything up. This was just whatever came to me to write about them. No matter how strange, I wrote it down.

When I was married, I never had what I thought that I had. What I had was created from an inauthentic me, and it came from a place of me trying to do what someone else thought I should do—and from me trying to be someone that I am not. What I had was created from a place of fear, fear of losing something I never really had anyway. It came from the fear of losing her, that dream woman, and the dream life that was promised.

Would she have stayed around if I had lived as me? Would she have stayed if I had just leaned into the fear and chosen myself over the deception of my mind? Who knows. But I would have had me all of those years, instead of a scared shell of me.

I was unhappy. I was living under the false adage of "happy wife, happy life." If you are living this way, start asking questions now! You and your family will be happy when you all choose to be happy, not because you make sacrifices in your life. Just to clarify: compromises ought to be reached when people who are being authentically themselves reach an agreement. Sacrifice, though, is when you let go of how you would do something only to please someone else. The other part of this is that the people in your life now get to make their choices based upon who you are and how you truly will choose for you.

I am not suggesting that you be what we consider selfish in this society (which is really self-centered, not selfish), just that you are authentically you from the get go, and all the way throughout any relationships you currently have, including that one with yourself and your life partner, your body.

This book will help you get into the frame of mind for this.

I didn't handle my affairs the way that my authentic self would have handled them. I did at first, and then was told that I was doing things incorrectly. I was told that I wasn't being a good protector and provider, even though I was handling things exactly how I would, and we were fine. But I began to doubt myself. Maybe I don't know how to do these things. Maybe I don't know really how to protect this woman, or earn money, or deal with clients...

I stopped doing things my way, and because I do a miserably poor job at doing things the way someone else would, I just stopped doing things out of fear of her reactions.

I stopped communicating about money because I was afraid of what she would say to me in return. This caused me to feel like I was wrong to focus on things that are kind of part of running your own small business. Combine that with being afraid of handling my business, my way, and I created a perfect storm. After enough time, she wandered away to look for someone who could provide a connection that was authentic, since I no longer provided that.

This caused me to then feel that the way I was, and would, run my business was wrong, and that the one thing that attracted people to my business — me -- was wrong.

Boom.

You see, when we operate on a platform that is anything less than uncompromisingly, un-authentically true to who we are, the world around us will provide exactly that in return.

Life is an echo of how we think and behave.

If we act authentically who we are, that is what we get back from the universe. We get that life that is authentically our life experience. It's when we stray from there either in thought or action (inaction) that we get the messy, not-so-fun stuff. The more we live our lives in this inauthentic way, the more of what we don't care for tends to build up.

What follows is doubt, disease, discomfort, unfulfilled dreams, weight gain, divorce, and even early death.

This preface has been the most difficult section of this book for me to write. But I feel that it tells the story of how I came to this project in a way that readers can hopefully connect with. I am no different than you. My journey, really, is no different. My ability to begin living my life by the questions, awareness, and principles laid out in these pages is by no means easier for me than it will be for you.

I still stumble. Writing this preface caused me to revisit all of the pain that sent me here. And I've had to utilize the tools in this book to keep my head about me. I can say that I feel clean having written this — as if getting this out has lifted something out of me, clearing the way for bliss to replace it.

Maybe writing your story down will help you as well?

What would that look like for you?

Who else might you help writing it down and sharing it?

This book is not a front to back story, nor is it an instructional manual that needs to be read in sequence. It is a collection of questions and awareness exercises that are to be used to ease the suffering in your life and lead into a state of what I like to call:

 Bliss in Embodiment—no matter what is going on in your world. I included practical applications, picked up over my 30-some years as an athlete, body builder, and personal trainer, which I compiled in chapter 4. As you read this book, your target is to relate the information back to your life and consider how it can help you!

Follow your Bliss - Greg Dyer

FOLLOW YOUR BLISS

If you follow your bliss, you put yourself on a kind of track that has been there all the while, waiting for you, and the life you ought to be living is the one you are living. Wherever you are – if you are following your bliss, you are enjoying that refreshment, that life within you, all the time.

– Joseph Campbell

Follow your Bliss - Greg Dyer

Introduction

It took me awhile to realize what it was that I was hearing — in fact it was about 45 years before I learned to listen and dance to the music. It's the music of the universe. And it speaks to us all. It just sounds different to everyone, and that's what makes this embodiment thing so interesting! Each of us is hearing the music and filtering it just a bit differently. So what happens when you wake up one day and begin to have the courage to share your music with the rest of us? This is what happened to me at 45 years old. I finally realized that what I was hearing wasn't just me making things up, but the music of the universe-the all-knowing thought that is there for all of us to tap into.

I call it the music of the universe because of my musical background: I've been writing and performing music as a drummer since I was 12. What I hear of the universal thought feels like the same source as the actual music that I hear, play, and produce. I write more about the music of the universe later on. What you are about to read here is me getting to explore these thoughts, the music of the universe, and sharing it with you all.

This all started innocently enough. I just started writing, noting observations of what was going on in front of me, distillations of things I have learned by reading others' work, my own practice as a body builder and personal trainer. I wrote newsletters and blogs. I have written things that I have never shared. Sometimes I "channel" things, meaning that I hear the thoughts and interpret them onto the page, very much like when I am writing music. It comes through me, not from me. This is the best writing, I feel. I don't have to force it — it just comes through. Like many others, I have felt a book coming through me for some time. The funny thing is, this isn't what I thought I would write! But here it is.

This is a collection of thoughts based on a single theme: achieving the most Bliss in Embodiment possible, in every moment, no matter what is going on. If you were to skim through this book and pick just one thought to read, pick the thought in chapter 2, Your Body: "What if weight gain is a symptom, not a problem to solve?" This one question and thoughts about it could flip the whole weight-loss industry upside down. Read it, and see how you look at the concept of weight gain and loss afterwards.

So what does it mean to follow your bliss anyway?

What if it were possible to have the most amount of fun, joy, happiness in this body, in this life of yours no matter what is going on? Whether things are going great, or maybe not so great? Fun, joy, and happiness whether you are in the throes of something you are passionate about or if you are just doing your taxes? (Well, I suppose someone out there likes doing taxes!) It is not only possible, but probable! It is just a matter of choice.

What does that mean, Greg — that it's a matter of choice? I know, it sounds like some unobtainable goal, reserved for those who choose to go live in a monastery, as far from civilization as possible. You get the concept, but the practice is just out of reach. Well, it really isn't. And I can show you how!

What if it is possible that we choose our lives and what happens in them? I know, there are an awful lot of bad things that happen to good people, but what if the sum total of our choices leads to where we are now? Not that we choose the awful things to happen, but that by not being mindful of the choices that we are making, the trail inevitably leads us here, to a place that isn't all that blissful, right? So this book is a collection of the thoughts, ideas, and channels I have read from others and applied for myself and for my clients. All of it leads to one place: more bliss in embodiment!

So what is embodiment anyway?

Embodiment is what you are doing right now. If you are reading this, you are here in this reality, inside an amazing body! Yes, I said "amazing"! And Beautiful, Wonderful, Spectacular!

Lesson number one towards Following Your Bliss: Start seeing your body and yourself as all of these things! Anything else is just judgment coming from sources other than Love, which is the language of the universe and (we'll talk more about this later).

A lot of the thoughts in this book have emerged during the last few years of my life — a time of change for me, and I imagine for more than a few of you all as well! It is just the nature of a life of impermanence. I know that I had been following most of these thoughts

all along, it was just that I had no other concept of life than that these thoughts belonged there. No matter what, I have been applying these thoughts in my life and seeing the results: more Bliss in Embodiment in my life!

So, who am I? How did I get to this point, to this way of thinking? To a point where I have a voice that contradicts the voice of nearly the entire fitness industry? When I was a body builder, I became a master at influencing my body's processes to do what I desired, which usually meant to carry as much muscle and as little fat as possible. I did it through awareness of how my body works, how it needed to do what I was asking, and by following through with those requests. I had had an interest in body building since my late teens. I was exposed to the sport by some friends at college who were pursuing it. I found the drive for muscle seductive, so I jumped in, training with them at first, following what they did, eating how they did, and taking supplements. I did it all not really knowing why, just that it felt good! I continued lifting on into my early twenties, then even gave a go at being a personal trainer when that service first became popular.

Life shifted for me, and I followed a fork that went into music. Playing drums in a rock band was a bigger dream, and I followed it. We gave it a good go, never quite reaching the level of sustainability, and by the end of my twenties, I found my way back to lifting weights. This time though, I had a focus that I never had when I was younger. I was driven. I eagerly gobbled up everything I could find on the subject! In two and a half years, I went from a couch potato to the body building stage, placing third in my first ever contest — and I loved it! I continued to learn everything I could, to apply the knowledge, weeding out what didn't work for me. Basically I turned myself into a lab rat, consuming everything I could find out about the sport, reading every article I could find to read — old school or new, it didn't matter. I desired to know everything I could, and how the pioneers of body building got to their levels was of particular interest. I wanted to know how it was possible to do so much with a lot less in the way of science. These guys just knew how to do it! The biggest take-away that from the whole experience for me was learning how I could manipulate my body and experiences by just believing and seeing that it was possible. Once I started, I never doubted that I could do it.

I started training my buddies in the gym and applying the knowledge I gained to guide them. It was working! The transformations that I saw were encouraging, and it wasn't too long after that when I turned it into a profession. At the urging of someone special in my life, the future mother of my daughter, I got certified as a Personal Trainer, picked a gym, and set up shop. I started applying what I learned about body building to my clients' lives, training them the same way I would train myself or another body builder. I quickly started questioning that process and started reading more about different methodologies, then applying those. What quickly became apparent to me was the fact that most of us in the training industry were using the same techniques we used to train body builders to train people who would never stand on stage as a body builder. It made no sense. Yet I saw it all over the place!

Why were we doing this? Training with body part splits (a different body part trained each day, so Monday would be chest, Tuesday back, Wednesday legs, etc.), going on fairly restrictive to totally restrictive diets that don't teach balance, just deprivation, and on and on? When all these people desired was just to get into shape, lose that extra weight, and be healthy. Why? What I found was this awareness: body building and the people who participated had been anointed to the epitome of what a healthy lifestyle and body are. Dangerously low body fat sometimes, along with ripped abs, arms, and chest!

This is an unrealistic pedestal for the people who do participate, and a poor measuring stick for what a body is supposed to look like. As a matter of fact, this is not at all what every body is supposed to look like, just some- just those who choose to engage in body building or some other sport that causes their bodies to look like that. It is not a measurement of a healthy body, a happy body, or a real body. It's just another example of what someone can accomplish here. It is not better or worse than your body, or anyone's body — it's just a different body.

Lesson number two towards Following Your Bliss: Stop comparing yourself and your body to others. Just stop! You are beautiful, amazing, and wonderful (see, we've circled back again to lesson number one). That uniqueness is needed here, because your unique experience is needed for the body and mind you have to experience this and for you to filter it all in your own amazing way. Share that experience with others! Abraham/Hicks

state that we are on the leading edge of thought right here, right in this reality[II]. Now knowing that, how else do we push that edge forward but by all of us sharing our unique experiences here in order to add to the collective and grow?

Now, I haven't always treated my body well. I am not 100 percent at it right now. I abuse it at times with food, too much sugar, and with too many carbohydrates. I do get out and spend time doing something I love physically, but not as much as I'd like. I do ride my bike when I can. It gives me bliss. The food thing can be bliss as well, and it is. I cook well and I love that — and I love to eat the food that I cook. This isn't the abuse, though. That relates to the quick sugars, muffins, chips, crackers, breads, and chai tea lattes in quantities that I feel are not always a contribution to bliss in embodiment. I think — no, I know, that this behavior is a result of feelings of failure, inadequacy, and a lack of worthiness. It is a way to fill the hole, so to speak. It is also a way to die. I asked for it. I asked to end this life after my wife separated from me.

I haven't really addressed this yet, until now, right here, with you reading this. I found this energy hanging about in my body, an ache deep within, growing into symptoms that I know will kill me if I leave them on this path.

We are going to clear this, you and I together. We are going to take all of this awareness that I have gathered over the years as a trainer, body builder, coach, and spiritualist, put it all together and guide ourselves into Bliss in Embodiment by Following Your Bliss.

What does that mean?

It is a space where we have the best time possible in these bodies, no matter what is going on. No matter what external or internal issues are happening, we are fully alive, conscious, aware, and engaged in the moment, and everything that the moment gives us. Do you know the general idea about happiness that is floating around out there? That somehow happiness is the end all, be all of existence? That we are supposed to somehow push all the negative thoughts and feelings out of our lives and just be happy?

Bull$#).*

That is not Bliss in Embodiment. That is denial. And BIE is not about denial. Bliss in Embodiment is about having the most connected experience that we can have, in every moment, no matter what is going on. I have to tell you something else: even when I was living the life of a body builder, eating clean, living clean, sleeping like I needed, working out in the gym regularly- doing all of the things that we are supposed to do to be healthy, I was still abusing this body. And I feel the reminders of that abuse pretty much every single day. So what about it? It is part of the Bliss, believe it or not!

I will explain: the extreme level which body building requires of participants to workout, diet, manipulate water and nutrients, deprive the body of what it needs to function properly, and use supplements and drugs to drop fat and water and build muscle creates an abusive environment for the body. When this goes on too long, just like anything else in life, it can create a chronic situation that may mean lasting effects on the body. Just as eating and drinking too much, becoming addicted to drugs and alcohol, or sex, anger, frustration, or depression, or sitting all the time.

So how could a choice to create that kind of experience with your body be blissful?

> *What we have is an amazing opportunity to be in bliss every day. To make choices to support bliss in embodiment, to choose to see the beauty in the life around us, causing that blissful feeling that is available at every moment. We have the chance to choose to not suffer from anything that may be happening to us that brings pain. Remember this: Pain is a chance to learn. Suffering is a choice to disconnect from bliss in embodiment.*

So what does that mean? We choose our type of suffering and how long we suffer. It is just a state of mind. You can choose to focus on the chronic pain in your back, knees, and neck, or on the diabetes, or any number of diseases we experience here. Or you can focus on the rest of life around you and on the beauty that surrounds us every day. We can focus on the fresh foods we have available to choose from and the taste experience we get from eating them. We can pay attention to the laughter of a child having fun — heck, we could join them. We can focus on the smell of a flower, the smell and feel of a loved one, the smell of coffee in the morning. On and on, the beauty of the experiences of life are all there for us to take in and enjoy.

When I choose to focus on these instead of on the reminders of injuries of past experiences in the gym, or other sporting endeavors when I may have pushed past my body's ability to tolerate, the suffering from the pain disappears. This goes for the sense of depression that comes from not being where you would like to be in life. No matter how that depression was created, taking time to engage in the beauty of the moment and focus on that instead of whatever it is that is causing the depression creates a sense of bliss in us.

Try it! Fully plug yourself into the moment right now and see how your body feels when you do. Notice your breath first. Inhale and exhale deeply into your belly a few times, noticing the feeling of your breath going in and out. See what else is there in the moment. Smells, tactile feelings. What are you hearing? Immerse yourself completely into the moment. Abandon your thoughts of past perceived failures and your worry about future issues. Just be here, right now. How does your body feel? How does your mind feel?

The more you do this, the better at it you get, and the cumulative effect is just like anything else that you do a little at a time. It's just like saving money in the bank: a little here and a little there adds up over time. Do this on a regular basis, and it adds up exponentially! There's no way to explain it—it just happens. Pretty soon, it is a habit, and you don't think about it.

You find your Bliss in Embodiment!

--Greg

Follow your Bliss - Greg Dyer

Chapter One

CONSCIOUSNESS

*Most people offer most of their vibrational offerings
in response to what they are observing, but there is no
creative control in that. Your creative control comes
only in deliberately offering thought -- and when you
are visualizing, you have complete control.*

-Abraham-Hicks

*You can do anything you want, if you put your mind to it.
It's just mind over matter.*

Light and Heavy

This is an Access Consciousness tool that is pretty useful, so I wanted to give it to you here. It is simple and goes like this:

The truth (your truth) will make you feel light. Lies (for you) will make you feel heavy.

This works for people every time. It's just a matter of learning what heavy and light feel like for you. With a little practice, you will have it down without thinking about it.

What would you use this for? You could use it for the type of movement you are picking to do, the type of foods you eat, or when and where to workout. The applications to the rest of your life are invaluable. Consider how you feel about the people with whom you are going to hang out? Would you really want to hang out with someone that causes you to feel heavy? This truth or lie is absolutely yours and yours alone. Check in with yourself if you feel heavy about a choice you are making. Ask yourself if it is really yours or someone else's?

Doubt

This life is teaching so many of us to look for the reasons why we can't do something. It's ingrained in us. Is it possibly a fear of succeeding on our own terms that keeps us from doing what we find blissful and exciting? Doing it our own way and being different than everyone else? Or, are we afraid of being ridiculed and judged for being different than others that holds us back? Is that really what the fear of success is?

So what happens then? Sometimes we just shut down completely, or do things half-assed. Or we just do things the way everyone else does them, because that is the way things are done. I've thought a lot about the times I have done just that in my life–done what others told me I should do, or how they told me to do it.

Quick story: I have played music and have wanted to be a musician for about as long as I can remember. That was all I wanted to do by the time I was a teenager. I was so sure that I would "make it." Then it came time to choose what to do after high school. I thought I was going to play music. Scratch that, I *knew* that I was going to play music! There was no way I was going to fail. I saw it in my mind. I saw the outcome via that mental map we make towards seeing our way to a goal, that motivation we use to do almost everything we succeed at in our lives.

Then came suggestions from others, and all were well-meaning suggestions for the most part, but usually they came out sounding something like, "Why don't you go to school and get a degree in something to fall back on in case it doesn't work out?" Some of them were a little more discouraging than that, but for the most part, well-meaning.

What did this do for me? It created a wedge of doubt in my mind. I ended up following the advice of the well-meaning suggestions and got a degree, then ended up having a 13- year career in the media. Good jobs, but not what I had planned for and saw in my mind. As you can guess, I never really "made it" as a musician. I never really gave it my all in my mind or in my actions. I always held back a little and deferred to the back-up plan.

Conversely, when I set out to do my first body building contest, I did do things my own way. I knew that if I did it that way, bucking the status quo of how to prepare for a contest, that I would achieve what I set out to do. And I did. I was successful at it!

What is the point that I am getting at here? This one question: What is holding you back from doing whatever it is that you would like to do your own way? Do you know why I ask this question? I ask it because it's only when you do things your own way, the way that you see in your mind and feel in your heart, that you will succeed at it. Sure, ask questions, seek out the guidance from those that have gone before, but never second guess or allow doubt to derail your vision of how you are going to succeed.

"Jump, and the net will be there."

Judging Our True Selves

What would it be like if we realized when we look at ourselves, or at others, that we are all together in oneness? We are all sharing a very similar experience here as human beings. We spend so much of our time judging our true selves out of existence. Think about that last phrase for a minute: Are you living as your true self, the one who is jumping around like a little kid inside of you, or are you living a life that you are "supposed" to be living to fit in with everyone else?

Whether it is what we say to ourselves in those deep, dark places in the recesses of our minds, or just outright to ourselves when we catch a glimpse of bodies in the mirror, we are almost always judging ourselves, deciding that we did that task wrong, that our bodies look wrong, that we made the wrong choice. How about what we say about others, and how we judge them for what they look like, how they act or speak? It always seems to be about the differences that we see from one another, or how different we may be from what is considered to be "normal" or "beautiful."

We can create what we would like here, you know. We can continue to live in the made- up world of the differences from each other, or the "ugly," "fat," "misshapen," too tall, too small, whatever "imperfection" bodies we inhabit, or we can ditch all of that and create a kinder life. We can create a life that realizes the similarities, the oneness we share, and celebrate our differences for what they are: a beautiful, unique, expression of humanity. We are each one-of-a-kind filters, here to contribute to the collective experience. It is really just a choice, and it can start with you.

When you wake up in the morning tomorrow, I want you to try thanking your body for the gift that it is to you, in whatever way you feel comfortable doing that. You can start off in your bed, just quietly saying, "Thank you, my body, for this amazing gift you give me, for this wonderful experience of life!" Try adding the words "You are beautiful" to the statement above. Notice how your body responds. When you feel comfortable with that, try looking at your body in the mirror and say the same thing. See if you can make this part of your daily routine.

When you catch yourself in a mirror during the day, reaffirm this statement. Start noticing what happens to the judgments of yourself, and for others as this practice becomes part of your routine. See what happens to your stress levels, your eating habits, and your sleep patterns. Notice how your body starts to change for you when you do this.

I think you are going to be surprised.

Living in the feeling

What does it mean to live in the feeling? Our feelings are what drive our entire experience here. Feelings are the channel for how we communicate with the universe, the path toward asking for what we would like to have in our lives. How that happens is really pretty cool. Knowing that it happens is powerful! We are conditioned in this reality to accept the role of a victim.

Yes we are!

Everything just happens to us, without too much participation on our parts. We lose our jobs, lose our spouses, catch colds, get cancer, have heart attacks, get a diabetes diagnosis. We get cut off in traffic, catch all the red lights, and the list goes on. Never once do we stop to consider the possibility that it is our energy, our feelings about ourselves and about the world around us that may be creating all of this.

Yes, all of this!

I know this is harsh to think about in the sense of things like, does someone really ask to be raped? Or do we really ask to be robbed or even murdered? Well, no. We don't. Well, not exactly anyway.

We do, however, harbor thoughts of inadequacy, of a lack of worthiness, and we have questions of our own lovability that when married to emotions of fears can create feelings of sadness, frustration, and anger that then broadcast those messages to the universe. The universe then goes about the process of sending similar energy to us — something that has the same or similar vibration to the feeling we are broadcasting out that support the feelings we are broadcasting. That is the Universe's job and it does this without prejudice.

If you allow yourself to be in this moment, not in the worry of the future, not in the anguish of the past, but right here in this moment, you offer yourself the possibilities to hear the awareness around you. This awareness may be quite different than what you have ever projected as possibilities for your life.

My question for you is this: Can you be in allowance for any and all of these possibilities to exist? Or are you stuck in a mode of my life, the next project, the lover I am waiting for, how much money I will make, and where it will come from must be a certain way? The universe gifts us back the things we have in our lives based upon feelings. The energy will match, but the specificity of things may not match exactly.

So, would you be able to allow for things to show up in different ways? Ways you may have never dreamed possible?

The language of the universe is our feelings. We are so conditioned to think our way through this life that we skip past the part that makes us successful when we do achieve success with something. When the moment arises that we get what we have been working, striving, hoping, and wishing for, we look past the obvious component that brought about that success. We congratulate ourselves for a job well done, we thank God for the blessing; we thank our parents, friends, bosses, fans for the help. But still we miss the easy part that caused the success. We look past the fact that we got a feeling involved in the process.

Think about the last time you succeeded at something: Did you not have the "feeling" that you couldn't fail at it? You just knew that it would happen for you. It's funny how we are so apt to look outside ourselves for the source of things that happen to us, good or bad. But what if you are the cause and the source of everything? Can you live with that? Or is it easier to believe that something else, someone else deserves the responsibility for everything?

Love

Love transcends all time and space. It is the bond that holds us all together, the language with which we speak to each other, around and beyond this reality. Even with all of the fear we throw at it, love remains intact, holding the balance of life. Amazing! It cannot be destroyed. Only in our minds, the minds of our egos, does fear have any chance of eclipsing love. Once beyond this reality, though, only a return to love awaits. It is a universal glue, a universal language.

Physicist Max Planck may have theorized of it in his findings of the space in between us, the space between everything, calling it the Matrix:

All matter originates and exists only by virtue of a force which brings the particle of an atom to vibration and holds this most minute solar system of the atom together. We must assume behind this force the existence of a conscious and intelligent mind. This mind is the matrix of all matter.[III]

Is it a stretch to theorize that this matrix may be love itself? Is it possible though that this space between everything, the stuff that science is working to understand and theorizes as dark matter and dark energy, is just what we feebly call love? Is it possible that we have such a limited view of things from here, that our perceptions of love are just a tiny part of it? That the stuff that makes up the in-between spaces is the unconditional, all-knowing connection to everything matrix that Max Planck suggested?

This energy is the glue, the source, the warm blanket if we desire to tap into it and pull it over us. It is our choice to tap into it, to listen to it, to wrap ourselves in it and utilize its all-knowing message from which we should conduct our lives. Is this all part of the unconditional love of the universe? I don't yet fully know, but does it hurt to conduct our

lives from this source? This is a question only you can answer. And there is no wrong answer, by the way. Just know that you have a choice, at all times. And you can re-choose anytime as well.

What would it mean to free ourselves from the tyranny of ourselves, to free ourselves from that oppressive feeling of no choice?

> I see the tyranny of ourselves as doubt– doubt in ourselves, the choices we make, and the thoughts that we have. Are the choices we make good enough? Are we good enough? Are we good enough for all of the amazing possibilities our minds can come up with for ourselves? Does it matter if these choices and thoughts align with what our family, friends, or society deems proper? The tyranny of ourselves (doubt) keeps us from what will ultimately be our Bliss in Embodiment.

Can you love yourself enough to drive the doubt out and connect to source more often? What would it feel like to operate from that space?

During a conversation with a friend about this, she brought up that deeper than doubt is fear. And most definitely fear can be the tyranny of ourselves.

The visionary scientist Gregg Braden says that there are only 2 emotions: love and whatever the culture you are from considers the opposite of love. For me, fear would be the opposite of love, so any feelings derived from that space opposite of love, like doubt, would derive from fear. I just like doubt in this instance. It seems a bit more to the point about how we sabotage ourselves. Besides, the awareness of doubt is what came through me while I was writing this. And since we are on the topic of the emotions of love and fear, and after the previous chapter about living in the feeling, how about an exercise to get into the space of communicating to the universe? This, by the way, is an exercise taught by Braden, and it is a powerful one!

Before we get into the exercise here, how about a little explanation of the chakra system, just so you have a road map of what I am explaining in the exercise to follow.

The chakras in Indian thought are the spiritual centers of the body. We have 7 basic chakras, 3 in the head, 4 in the body. They are in order from the bottom up:

1. **Root Chakra** — Represents our foundation and feeling of being grounded.

    - **Location:** Base of spine in tailbone area.
    - **Emotional issues:** Survival issues such as financial independence, money, food.

2. **Sacral Chakra** — Represents our connection and ability to accept others and new experiences.

    - **Location:** Lower abdomen, about 2 inches below the navel and 2 inches in.

- **Emotional issues:** Sense of abundance, well-being, pleasure, sexuality.

3. **Solar Plexus Chakra** — Represents our ability to be confident and in control of our lives.

    - **Location:** Upper abdomen in the stomach area.
    - **Emotional issues:** Self-worth, self-confidence, self-esteem.

4. **Heart Chakra** — Represents our ability to love.

    - **Location:** Center of chest just above the heart.
    - **Emotional issues:** Love, joy, inner peace.

5. **Throat Chakra** — Represents our ability to communicate.

    - **Location:** Throat.
    - **Emotional issues:** Communication, self-expression of feelings and the truth.

6. **Third Eye Chakra** — Represents our ability to focus on and see the big picture.

    - **Location:** Forehead between the eyes (also called the Brow Chakra).
    - **Emotional issues:** Intuition, imagination, wisdom, the ability to think and make decisions.

7. **Crown Chakra** — Represents our ability to be fully connected spiritually (the highest chakra).

    - **Location:** The very top of the head.
    - **Emotional issues:** Inner and outer beauty, our connection to spirituality and pure bliss.[IV]
    - On to the exercise then!

So think of the thoughts in your head as kind of originating in between your crown chakra and the next on down your third eye chakra, and your emotions originating from your root chakra (down in your pelvis area).

For this exercise, you can take whatever thought that you have. It could be a thought about getting a new job, for example. Take this thought and marry it with one of the 2 emotions, love or fear. The energy of this meets in the middle, in your heart chakra, which creates the feelings associated with the thought. So consider the thought of bringing a special person into your life. Maybe there is a programmed sense of fear associated with the thought, a fear of that never happening for you. We marry these together in the middle, in the heart, and a feeling is created for it — a feeling of sadness, dread, or depression.

Now for the powerful part of this: This is the energetic language of the universe. This is how we speak out for what we want. So these feelings of sadness and depression attract a like energy, a near affirmation from the universe for what it is you are asking for, like the feeling that you will never attract that special person to your life. And so it is then.

So what happens if you take that original thought of desiring that a special person shows up in your life and you marry it instead with love, shifting yourself out of that pattern of meeting your thoughts with fear? What feelings now show up in your heart?

Try it. See what you get.

Most of us have an internal dialogue, or predominant thought pattern that just runs on auto-pilot in the background, so adjusting this pattern with some conscious work on your thought patterns could be the next trick for you. In the back of this book on p.120, I have included an exercise to adjust your background dialogue.

What would it look like to just embrace change?

It is going to happen regardless of our allowance or participation. When I look back on the 3 decades of "adult" life that I have experienced, all I see is a constancy of change. I was reflecting on the last 6 years specifically, noticing that at that time, 6 years ago, I was living with my now ex-wife, with a brand new baby, playing in a rock band and recording my own music in the studio that I built in the basement of the house we bought together. I was training people, but I hadn't yet to put together the consciousness part of it, the mind-body connection.

Fast-forward to present day: I am divorced, and I lived in a room at a friend house during this transition, sharing it about half the week with my now 6-year-old daughter. I don't play music anymore; as a matter of fact, I really don't even own my drums anymore. I pawned them for money to live on. I now live in a nice one bedroom-plus-study townhome after spending about 6 months of this transition in a kind of dodgy one- bedroom apartment that forced me to move out because of a mold problem!

I no longer write music either. I've sold off much of the studio equipment I cobbled together over a decade as well. But, the shift in my business world is the most amazing! Having embraced the mind-body approach to things, I have found a path I never saw before. The thing that allowed me to see it was finally embracing the changes that were going on and then finding something to create. As I created, I attracted more possibilities into my life. As I choose the possibilities that looked fun to do, I attracted more of the same type of energy. People started showing up that are willing to be part of what I am creating. I am getting help! It is amazing and magical! Part of it, well, a big part of it was my willingness to embrace being uncomfortable.

To be honest, being comfortable is where dreams go to die. Making the move to get out of the rut I was in became really uncomfortable! What I found was a requirement for me at least to start creating, and creating for me at the time was to write. I went up to the mountains on the weekend and just wrote for hours. I would head to coffee shops after an evening training people and just write until the shop closed.

It started out as just writing the awareness that came to me about questions I had asked and put on sticky notes. What it became was therapy. It also became Conscious. Body. Movement. I began creating something beyond what was comfortable for me. I began to

bounce out of the rut. I really struggled at times with the validity of what I was doing, questioning whether a personal trainer, me specifically, really had what it took to do this. Was what I was writing really worth anything? Was I worthy of creating something like this? Who was I to be so audacious to think that I could bring consciousness to the world? I had no formal education in anything related to the topic. I am not a doctor or PhD of anything! I make my living as a personal trainer.

It turns out that the more I wrote, the more I shot videos of my awareness, and the more I talked to people, the more confidence I gained. The more questions I asked, the less I really cared about what anyone thought about what I was doing- and the more I found people interested in what I am doing.

As for the people that aren't interested, or think I am crazy? Well, they are kind of moving on. Things are changing. Some of it changed without my active participation, meaning, I didn't make a conscious choice to have it changed. But it changed anyway. What do I do with that now? I could go into the wrongness of me. I could do the "woulda, coulda, shoulda" game. I could lament over the loss of something I thought I would have the rest of my life. Guess what? I did some of all of that. I rolled around in that slop like a pig in poop. Only I wasn't happy. Where I found the tiny rays of happiness was in the writing, shooting videos, in sharing my thoughts- the creating. It carried over into the gym. I began enjoying training people again. I attracted new clients that really were looking for the way that I do things.

As I grew into this newness for me, I found something else, someone else that was right there under my nose. A friend became more than that. I found someone who was travelling the same path as I was and asking the same kind of questions, creating a similar life. And the joy that comes from sharing time with her is re-lighting things for me. It is having a calming effect, which causes me to be still and to "hear" more awareness. Along with the questions I still ask, I am finding something far more powerful than the question. It is a knowing.

This knowing is the space that pushes doubt completely out of my head. You have it too.

The Speed of Choice

What is the speed of choice?

It is the idea that everything comes to us once we make the choice for it. How that happens is up to the universe, and it's up to us to be able to receive that which is coming from the universe. It is likely that it will show up in a way that is unrecognizable to us and our concepts based upon judgment. You see, we have conclusion built into our system here. Things must show up for us only in the ways that make sense to us, ways that we have been taught for them to happen.

A+B=C. If you do this, then that will happen.

There is always a sense that things must happen for us after we work for them, struggle

for them. If things show up any other way, and we happen to recognize them, to receive them that way is a struggle in itself, requiring us to let go of this reality's sense of right and wrong. So the speed of choice actually, ironically, has its own requirement. It is that you must be willing to be in reception of everything, any way that it may come? How do we do that?

We do it through vulnerability. This isn't this reality's sense of that term. We have bastardized it into a pejorative term. But true vulnerability is strength. It is an awareness of all that is around you. It is like sinking into a warm bath and sensing all that the bath has to offer you. It is like being in the womb again, and knowing you are safe no matter what.

So how does this relate to the speed of choice? When we remove the requirement to judge all, to conclude how things may come to us, we can become more vulnerable. This vulnerability now gives us the ability to receive all of the awareness around us. So no matter how the universe may gift us, we can be available to receive it. Once we make the choice to be vulnerable, we leave ourselves open to receive. This is a scary concept for most, because it is generally perceived that being that open leaves us in a position to be taken advantage of, or in a position to be hurt. That is not being vulnerable. That is setting yourself up to be a victim by not being open for all of the awareness around you. It is ignorance and egoism that sets us up to be hurt, not vulnerability.

So things happening to us in the speed of choice are related only to us making the choice to not judge an outcome, in us having no vested interest in what may be. It happens by just letting go of any expectations. Can you do it? What if it were to become an everyday practice? Just like anything else we learn to do, we consciously make the choice to do this. After a while it becomes second-nature. We no longer have to think about doing it. How?

Start with 2 things:

Practice gratitude for everything in your life– all of it, even the stuff you have judged as "bad" (see, there's s that letting go of judgment thing). Next time someone pays you a compliment or gives you a gift, just say thank you. No qualifiers, no sense of debt in the receiving of the gift, no mention of worthiness for it, i.e., "Oh you shouldn't have! That is too expensive." That is not receiving: That is speaking to your worthiness of the gift. And if you are the giver, no gifting with the thought of building some kind of gift equity there. The unadulterated reception of your gift is the return of that gift energy.

Resistance

There is something so fundamental about unwanted weight gain, pain, and disease.

(For now, let's put them all under dis-ease.) It is lifestyle choice, but why do we make those choices? It is a resistance to something. Find what is being resisted, and we unravel the thread, the choices that lead to the dis-ease. Who do we really be? Who is looking back at you in the mirror? Is it someone you recognize? Is there any part to that image in the mirror that you do not recognize?

This is where we start to find out just what is being resisted. Because that is the mask we – you – put on to hide a truth about you that you are avoiding or resisting. Why are you resisting? Can you be honest with yourself? It doesn't even matter if you are honest with others; the honesty/dishonesty with yourself forms the basis of choices (the ones that drive your lifestyle, supply your life with bliss or no bliss) from which you create.

Choosing Happiness

I recently read an article that caused me to think about this. It was about all of the things that supposedly if we had, we would be happy, including a flat, washboard stomach, a good marriage, a dream job, money, new car, a house, and on and on. Every day I hear people speak about these things, especially in the gym. I'll hear things like, "If I could just lose the last 2 pounds, I'll be happy!" Really?

I want to tell you all something: I have had washboard abs. *Several times in my life.* I have met and married the *right* woman… twice. I have had the truck of my dreams.

I have had a house of my own (shared with my family). On that note, I have had an intact family. I have had more than enough money to live on. I spent it. I have had savings. I spent it. I've been on trips to exotic places. I've had best friends.

How much happiness did all of that get me really? Nothing. Nada. Zip. None of those things brought me happiness, at least not anything more that temporary and superficial.

Was I happy with those things and those people? Yes. But those things and those people did not bring me happiness. Am I happy now? That depends. On what, you ask? On whether or not I am choosing happiness in the moment. And what exactly is choosing happiness in the moment?

If you can find yourself paying attention to the moment, not worried about the future, or feeling guilty about something from the past, you can find yourself happy. It's an exercise at first, something you consciously choose to do. Eventually it will settle into your subconscious routines and become "second nature."

I have also found that I become a master of time when I do this. So not only do I find myself blissfully happy, I slow time down as well, making the experiences last longer!

Another part of this is to find yourself grateful for the moment, and for everything and everyone in your life. After all, you have brought them there. Why else would you choose something or someone in your life, except that somewhere in your world you desired that? Think about it. Where are you right now in your mind?

Are you here, in the moment?

We All Have Our Stories

We all have our stories, the stories we tell ourselves of how our life is, how it will be.

We also tell stories of what is happening. Sometimes they match with what we are telling ourselves, sometime they don't. Does it really matter if the stories match up? It is, after all, your life. Create it how you see fit.

What I would like to bring up here is this: what effect do our stories have on our bodies and our communion with our bodies? You see, our bodies are like a reflection of what we think about ourselves and about our lives. As such, our bodies will show us and the rest of the world just what is going on inside our heads.

Awareness came to me some time ago that our perceptions of ourselves equals our projection of ourselves. Thoughts will project through the body. It tells a story too. It tells your story, the one you may be living, the one you may be hiding from yourself, and maybe from the rest of the world out of fear of judgment. It may be telling about a life you are living that is not your own.

So then, what does that story you are living, the one that is not yours, tell your body or tell the rest of the world? Good question, huh? What would it take to connect with that story? What would it take to connect with the story that *is* yours? If you know that you are living a story that isn't yours, can you remember when you adopted this story and why? Is there a purpose to living this story? Does it feed something else for you, or are you afraid to step into your story? What is holding you back? Are you afraid of losing something or somebody? Is this worth not living your story?

When you have the awareness of what or who is holding you back and if it is worth living some other story than yours, you will begin the path towards creating your true story.

You may not lose what you think you are going to lose. But I can assure you, what you will gain by living your story has the possibility to bring you more than you can imagine.

How will this affect your body?

I ask you this: when you are absorbed in the moment doing something you love to do, how does your body feel? How, then, do you think you will feel living your story every minute of every day? What is holding you back?

Go for it!

The Compass

There is a space inside us. It is a space where the entire path that can lie before us resides.

It is a compass of sorts, guiding us along the way. We can choose to follow it or not. It is entirely up to us. This compass creates the need for change. Sometimes that change just goes about its way, independent of us. The compass and its path are a powerful force in our lives. Resistance to any change can create its own energy, its own change. It can manifest in pain for us. This can be emotional, physical, or spiritual pain. This is part of the compass' job as well. It is kind of like the feeling of getting kicked out of the nest. It is time to grow into the next greatness of you– not necessarily leaving the past behind, but no longer living there.

The past was yours. It was what you did. But it did not make you who you are; you and your choices have done that. Take your personal power back, and know your ability to create your world. The past was just the compass' guidance, the choices you made to follow or to not follow what the compass was showing you. If you are in pain, there is a question to ask yourself: Where am I resisting the guidance the compass is showing me?

What would happen if you followed that awareness?

You Can't Stay Here Anymore

Have you ever had that wonky energy feeling, either with a friend, loved one, job, place you live, or yourself? Has it been creating a sense of ill in your body, possibly even creating disease? The desire to eat more to fill a hole left in you, or to mask a pain? Has it caused you to just run away or hide? Well, what other possibilities are there for you?

Is it possible that this feeling is a sense of the universe, or God, telling you that it is time to step into more greatness of you? You can't stay where you are at forever. This is one of the constants of the universe and of our lives: change. Can you answer the call? Many of you are probably saying, "I feel this, but I don't know where to go!" Well, what if you do? What if you look inside yourself, into that spot that holds your greatest desires? What do you feel and see there? What if that is where you are being guided to go? What would it take to step towards that?

Take the next step and see what happens after that. It most likely is the uncomfortable step that you are avoiding to take-- the one step that causes you some trepidation and pause. Maybe you have been putting it off for some time. I personally found that when I lean into, or step into, this greatness for me, no matter how uncomfortable it feels, my aches and pains in my body just disappear! My weight drops down, and I feel invincible, full of energy and vitality, and I feel happiest!

So what can you step into today to begin leaving where you are now? Because you don't have to go home, but you can't stay here!

Can You Hear the Music?

There is a revolution upon us. It is not coming- it is upon us now. It is a revolution of thought. We are just trying like hell to avoid it, to postpone the inevitable shift that is here within all of us. We are trying to avoid that voice in our heads, no matter how buried, shouting that this reality we are living is not enough, not what we signed on for, not our higher callings.

Is it a possibility that the strife that we feel, the fighting, the struggle with one another is this knowing within ourselves that settling for the status quo of what this reality offers is not enough? And is this "hiding" of our true gifts, our true voice, the music that plays inside us (which so many of us so often just completely ignore), part of or the whole of this discontent that we feel?

We are hiding ourselves and our music from the world because of the judgment we face from others about being different. This transfers to us as a judgment on our own thoughts and actions. We are creating our lives from judgment. This simply must stop.

Until we stop this, we will never create the amazing life we are capable of. Judgment is an illusion. That is all. It has nothing to do with our truth. Our music is not created from judgment. Judgment can only serve to dampen or put out entirely the fires that burn within us. Accepting judgment is not acting in service to one another.

There is a truth that rings loud and clear about being in service of others. This concept was difficult for me to get until just recently. I thought that being in service to another was giving of one's time to help another — to completely ignore what it is that you have to offer the world, to ignore your story, your gift in favor of helping someone else who is struggling. I believed that somehow the people selflessly giving of themselves, despite their own wishes, were the only ones living in service of others, and if we didn't give of ourselves to others, then we were being selfish.

Well, these notions are rooted in judgment. We are in service to others when we live our truth, when we allow our music to come out to the world. It is a disservice to the world to "die with your music within you"! To do our own thing, without judgment of ourselves, and to ignore the judgment of others- that is our gift to the world. That is living in service to others.

We are on the cutting edge of thought here. We are the creators of this reality. Our voice is so much of the overall story of this, and we have done such an amazing job of almost wiping this out in favor of fitting in!

Well, enough. That is enough for me, enough for you, enough of teaching our children to squash their stories, their dreams, in favor of "fitting in."

I have loved one line from the movie *Brave Heart* more than any other line or quote:

"Your heart is free. Have the courage to follow it." You, me, all of us: It is time to live our lives by this mantra. This is revolution that I am speaking of.

I am here to free all of those who want to come with me from the shackles that this reality has put upon us. They are not really there. We just keep telling the stories so often and with so much conviction that we have made the bonds real. Why do I think I am so special? That I am the one to free us from this? Because, this is my music! This is what I hear from Source, God, the universe, whatever you wish to call it. I am special. Yes. But guess what? So are you. And I am here to show you that, just as I show myself that. I don't mean this in some kumbaya sort of way, that free love, "we are all special" crap. I mean it in that it is time to let all of the bull$&*7, oppressive thought patterns that this reality is putting upon us — no, that *we* are allowing to be put upon us — to disappear.

You are special. You are needed. *Your* contribution is required NOW!

It is time for all of us to get off of our butts and get after it! Let your dreams, your voice, out into the world! There is something that I have recently started telling my clients that I would like to share with you. The potential judgment that you face from others for doing your thing is so much more fun than the pain you will feel from keeping that inside. I know this to be truth. I've been married twice now, to 2 different women. yes. Trust me when I say I have had a bunch of judgment for myself for this. I still do from time to time. That has proven to be nothing but a waste of my imagination. That judgment has done nothing for me but pull my energy down so far that I couldn't hear the music any more.

Another part of this story is what was happening while I was married to these 2 women. The judgment that I was allowing to affect me from both of them also was pulling my energy down so I couldn't hear the music. We are doing this to ourselves, to one another, every day. This only serves to pull our energies down far enough that we can't hear the music anymore. This is what judgment does.

Now, there are many examples throughout history, and with us all the time, of people who have cut through the haze of judgment, not allowing it to affect them or take them down enough so that they couldn't hear their music anymore. These are the thought leaders. These are the ones that push through to let their music out to the world, regardless and in spite of the judgment thrown at them from loved ones, peers, or "authority figures."

They know beyond a doubt that what they hear must come out of their head, their mind—that great filtering device we have between our ears—and become a contribution to the world. Our minds are a gift. They filter the music we hear into our unique voice. This is what makes us, you and me, special, that unique way of hearing the music that is going on all the time. The music is the inspiration from the universe.

This revolution that I am writing about is us reaching a tipping point. More and more people are letting go of the hold that judgment has and letting their voices speak.

What happens if all of us do just that? What happens when we teach—no show, our children that not only is it okay to be different, to have different thoughts, but that it is actually mandatory? It is judgment that keeps us down. Judgment keeps us in lower vibrations so we can't hear the music. All of the judgment of ourselves, our allowance of judgment from others, the fear of being judged out of being needed, wanted, and the fear of not fitting in is keeping us down in lower vibratory patterns.

There is a really cool thing that happens when we step out of the shadows of judgment and let our music out: The people that are attracted to that music show up to support our efforts to let that music out! And the ones that are not attracted to it, the ones who want to judge you out of that effort, will either begin to see what you are doing and drop the judgment of you, or they will just disappear from your life. Both are okay results. Both work out in your favor. And what if by doing your thing, letting your music out to the world, inspires others? What if you can inspire those who are trying to judge you out of dancing to your music to just ignore the judgment and do their own thing too?

What if all the agreements we have made with our lives could be renegotiated, or let go of?

What could this offer as possibility now, if everything that you have decided was going to happen for you, to you, with you, if every agreement you have made with yourself or someone else could be renegotiated or let go of all together?

Could you start over? Could you just do something different?

And if you could do this (and you can) what would you do differently? What would you choose for yourself?

You may be asking what this series of questions has to do with your body and what is possible with it — weight loss, muscle/strength gain, flexibility, aerobic capacity. Well, our thoughts and choices influence what our bodies will do for us. If we are making choices that are out of alignment with who we could be, they can and do show up in the body as dis-ease.

How does it get any better than that — that sometimes a choice that was once in alignment of who we are (but is no longer) just comes to an end?

We keep going based on familiar patterns, or we just do so because we are supposed to do things that way. But what if you could choose any possibility, at any moment of your life, as often as you would like?

How do you suppose your body would respond to you choosing for you?

This judgment of your body: does it belong to you or someone else?

This will work with any judgment, but let's look at your body for this example. First off, another question: If it were just you here, no one else, no media, no friends or family, to whom would you compare yourself in order to get those judgments of yourself?

So what if you operated as if you are the only one here when it comes to the judgments you place upon your body?

Those judgments, do they belong to you anyway?

I've been told that something like 98 percent of the thoughts in our head don't belong to us anyway. Ask yourself why you would choose to judge your body in an unkind manner.

The next time one of these unkind thoughts pops up, ask yourself, does this thought really belong to me, or is it someone else's? Do you feel lighter when you ask that question? It's probably not your thought, which means it didn't originate from your head. You picked it up from somewhere else, or from someone else.

Try this: Just say I return this thought to sender with consciousness.

Just see how you feel after doing that.

What if your body creates itself from the judgments you have of it?

If all you heard all the time was how dumb you were, what would you create for yourself?

What would you believe after a while? That you are dumb? What do you think is possible with what you tell your body about it?

If you are constantly calling your body fat, ugly, too short, too tall, too dark, too light, or something like that, how does your body respond to that? Or, how do you and your body work together to create that as a reality?

How does that create what you see?

Here's another way to think about this: Would you say the things you are saying to your body to your best friend, your lover, a family member, or anyone else for that matter?

Why say them to your own body then?

So how can you reframe those thoughts about your body? At the end of the book on p. 120 is an exercise to go through to reframe your dominant thoughts. This can be used to reframe your thoughts about your body as well.

But know this: You and your body are spectacular, wonderful, beautiful, amazing, magical, and infinite just as you are now. The people that are worthy of having in your life know this and see it. The ones who see something different and choose to judge you are themselves dealing with some other issue and you don't require them around all the time, do you?

And if they are part of your life on a daily, weekly, monthly basis, how can you choose to not be the sum total effect of their opinions of you, which causes you to adopt their opinion of you and your body?

If they are part of your life in a capacity that is closer than, say, a co-worker, do you really require them to be that close? And one other thought about this: What if you held the opinion of yourself and of your body that you are both beautiful? How would others see us if we taught them how to treat us?

What if there is nothing wrong with you?

What if all the choices you make are just that, choices?

These choices can be re-chosen, or you can choose differently at any time! What energy does it bring to accuse yourself of being wrong for a choice made?

Does it feel heavy or light to accuse yourself of being wrong?

Knowing that it was just a choice — nothing else — know that you can choose again. In any 10 seconds! You can use that experience to know that, well, you just tried something in a way that won't work for you. And how can it get any better than to become aware of something that doesn't work for you?

It can just be data for your life.

Another part of this to consider: Do those thoughts of wrongness belong to you, or to someone else? Since somewhere around 98 percent of the thoughts in our heads don't even belong to us, they must come from all around us, from the people with whom we are in close contact, and even the ones that share this planet with us! It may sound strange, but we are like psychic antennae, picking up the broadcasts of thousands and thousands of signals from others around us.

With about 95 percent of the people walking around having the thoughts of wrongness of one kind or another, this is a good question to ask: Does this belong to me or to someone else? Dr. Dain Heer of Access Consciousness has suggested doing this for 3 to 5 days straight and feeling the weight of that negative self talk drop away.

To whom does that wrongness you feel about the food you eat, the size of your clothes, whether or not you go to the gym, or what you look like really belong to? If you were just you, would you really be that unkind to yourself and your body?

What if you didn't have to have a sense of purpose?

So much importance is placed on a sense of purpose, what we do in life, like it is all that we are. If you don't do the "right" things (go to school, get a good job, find the right boy/girl, get married, have kids, the right house in the right neighborhood, put the kids in the right school, vacation in the right places, and the list goes on and on), your sense of purpose is judged as wrong. What is that all about? Are you living your life or everyone else's life?

So what would happen if you didn't have a sense of purpose: Could you more freely choose anything, in any given moment? If you were not defined by your sense of purpose, who are you? Who could you now be? Could you shift to handle any given situation with more ease if you weren't busy defining yourself?

If you define yourself based on societal ideals, what happens to the person that you truly could be if that didn't align with society's ideals? What can happen now in your body if that energy is ignored, stuffed down, or given up on all together? Would your body reflect that discomfort in your soul? Dis-ease maybe? Weight gain?

So if you shifted into no definition, no sense of purpose (which by the way doesn't mean you do nothing, just that the definitions of life can be changed in any given moment), how would that affect your body now?

If you choose for yourself in any given moment, free from the constraints of purpose, what would you choose and create for yourself and for your body in this moment?

What if we let go of expectation of how life should be?

So what would your life be like without the expectations of what is to come? Would you be more available for the present?

What if with the projections of expectation comes the equal chance of great joy and great disappointment? What would you do with that awareness when you are putting expectations on your life? With the disappointments come the possibilities of them building up, creating a depression.

What if that depression is asking to be fed? Are your food choices feeding depression?

Psst... You have choices!

What if you keep it to once a day?

I know you have something you really like to eat or drink. So you reach for this often throughout the day. It could be diet soda, cookies, chips, candy, or Starbucks — anything you enjoy several times a day. It becomes a habit for you, which is fine. No wrongness here. Just ask yourself this question: Has this habit become an unconscious one?

This can be contributing to the extra fat you have gained and the fat you continue to gain. As a trainer, I have seen this over and over again. If a person were to just stop the diet soda, he or she could drop at least 10 pounds in a month, with no change other than that! I have this question for you, because I really don't care for total deprivation when it comes to dieting: What if you had just one a day? Whatever that may be, restrict yourself to one. This can take care of the desire to have it, while reducing the detrimental effects of having multiples. So what if you gave "once a day" a try and see what happens for you?

It really is that easy?!

It can't be, right? It can't be that easy to lose weight, get into shape, to do anything you want to with your body. It requires hard work, discipline, and effort, right?

What if it isn't hard work, discipline, or effort that makes it possible, but instead choice? What if it is just simply that somewhere, in some way, you are failing to choose this to happen?

I can hear the wheels spinning now! Some of you have gone into "there is no way that that is possible" mode. I just need to knuckle down and get it done! Others of you just went to "what is wrong with me that I just can't seem to choose it" mode. Well, I have something for all of you, no matter where you went just then. What if the reason you are not choosing the path that you think you have chosen has to do with it not being your path?

Huh? Come again?

Read that again: What if the reason you are not choosing the path that you think you have chosen has to do with it not being your path? What would that mean to you? What if there is another way that you and your body would like to lose weight?

What if the way that you have "adopted" is just not the way you will do it? It doesn't float your boat, so to speak. And if it is something that isn't yours, the possibilities of you succeeding with it are slim to none. Just because Mr. or Ms. Perfect has success with this program you want to do, does not guarantee your success! What you will have success with is what your bliss is! This is the movement or exercise that you will do because it is fun! This will be the way to eat for you because it is easy and fun for you.

With that, the hard work becomes fun! The discipline is something that is just part of you, like sitting on the couch and watching TV. And the effort will feel more like play, and just like that. It really is that easy!

What if all the knowledge of how it is supposed to happen is getting in the way of it happening?

You have done all the research, asked a bunch of questions, and prepared a detailed plan for how you are going to lose weight. Great! You have been religiously following said plan for a few months now and you've lost a few pounds. Cool! But it's not happening nearly as fast as you would like. The weight just isn't coming off that quickly. What gives? All the "experts" have been consulted; this is a tried and tested program! It should work, damn it! But it isn't, huh?

What if all of that knowledge you have amassed to create the perfect program has actually blocked the awareness of how your body would really like to do this?

Huh?

You have created THE way this is going to work! No need for any superfluous information, right? That will only get in the way and confuse things, right? But what if that superfluous information is feedback your body is giving you on what it would like from you?

Yes, it may not be coming from your body; it may be an article that showed up, a person with another idea, or just some random bit that fell into your head. But you discarded it, right? Because you have THE plan! By being locked into one way of doing things, you may be ignoring something that actually might help you.

So what to do?

What if you used your awareness about this? I am not suggesting that you hop from plan to plan to plan, willy nilly. That is not being aware or conscious. That is just hopping from shiny new object to shiny new object. That has never worked. Listen to the information coming into your awareness as you proceed. If something feels right, feels right for you, what would happen if you used it to guide your way? What if you weren't afraid to do that?

Ask questions! Keep asking questions, even when things are going well in your fat loss plan. It's been said that the answers lie in the details. What if the details lie in the questions?

You are "perfect" the way you are!

What if you already know this? And that all that internal dialog telling you that you are not perfect doesn't even belong to you?

Let me ask you a question: Would you really be so unkind to yourself as to continuously beat yourself up for being less than perfect? And who are you comparing yourself to anyway?

Think about this the next time you are comparing yourself to someone else: Are you comparing you at your perceived worst to someone else's perceived best? How could that ever work for any of us? How could you ever measure up in that instance if you are comparing?

What if you just didn't compare yourself to anyone else? Who else can be YOU better than you? And can you really be someone else?

So what would all this comparing lead to other than disappointment?

You are unique, amazing, special, beautiful, and magical! And you do know this. Don't you?

Deep down, it's there. Look inside. Look down where you put stuff that doesn't fit into this reality. It's there. Your confidence is there—the confidence in knowing you are perfect just the way you are!

So next time you see something on TV or in print that tells you that you are less than perfect, that unless you do things a certain way, buy a certain product, or look a certain way, know this: *That is a manipulation to get you to follow an agenda that does not belong to you!* I am not suggesting that you are wrong if you do, just letting you know that you have a choice here. You have the choice to follow the agenda or to carve out your own path, knowing full well that you and only you can do you perfectly.

Validating Trauma and Drama

This trauma and drama thing is the way we measure our lives, our worthiness, and our progress, at least in this reality. But what if we don't really need those? What if it is just a choice for us to use them? And what does it mean to validate trauma and drama?

Think about this in your life: How are we with others around us? If something traumatic or dramatic like illness, divorce, or a death happens in our lives, what do those who care do for us? Or to be more precise, what do they do to us?

Have you used this one, or heard it before? "Oh, you poor baby, things will get better!" Or, "That is such a tragedy. You poor thing!"

What do those words do for us? They validate the event, they validate the trauma or drama! They can set it into stone, so that now all it can ever be is that traumatic or dramatic event. Well, what else could it be, you ask?

Nothing if we accept the event as something traumatic.

Is it possible, though, that pain is an inevitability of our lives, but suffering is a choice? And does the validation of the trauma and drama perpetuate that suffering?

But Greg, you say, by relating those things to our friends and loved ones, we show that we care! Maybe, but what if there were another way? What if we instead ask what we can offer as help? What does that person require to lessen the impact of the event?

So instead of validating that person's suffering in and around the event, we offer assistance out of it?

And on the flip side of that, what if when a traumatic or dramatic event happens to you, and when someone then offers up one of those validating statements, you just return that judgment right back to sender—or you say to yourself that it is just an interesting point of view?

What if you then had the courage to ask for what you may really require from that person, in that moment, in lieu of the validating statement?

Beyond that, what if you just chose to view life events not as traumatic or dramatic, but just as additional experiences that demonstrate for you ways that won't work for you, or as things that sometimes just happen in life, and then you choose to move on?

Another question for you: What if the validation of the trauma and drama is causing your body to go into protection mode and to store fat?

*What could be happening to your body as
you validate trauma and drama?*

What is actually happening in your body as you go through trauma and drama? You probably know that these are stresses, but what could this stress be telling your body to do?

Is it at all possible that your body could sense this chronic stress as a need to protect you? Check in with yourself to see if this feels light or right. So what could happen in this protection mode? There are a couple of things that your body can do for you that are really quite cool! Yes, I said "do *for* you." Your body will protect you from perceived stresses. There are 2 possibilities that this breaks down to as far as the body is concerned:

Get skinny so to be able to out run a threat of being eaten, or, put on body fat to protect from the body from cold or famine. Today's daily stresses aren't quite the same, but there exist more stresses now than ever in the history of mankind! Still, our bodies are wired pretty much the same way as they have been for 100,000-plus years.

Today's stresses can be interpreted by the body as a threat as I mentioned above, thus causing the body to speed up the metabolism, or to slow it down. Which direction that goes is different per each individual, though. What may cause one person to get skinny can cause another to put on fat. What can you do about it? The simple answer is to remove the stress and tell the body that you are safe.

But how do we do that? Move to the mountains and become a hermit, duh. Well, that might work, but what could be some more practical ways? Maybe it's a change in jobs, or a change in where you live. Maybe it's removing yourself from an abusive situation. Meditation is a great form of stress relief, as is physical exercise.

I have a question to leave you with though: What is it inside you that you feel you be, that you are not being? (Throughout this book I will use the verb be instead of are, as in "you be". I use this for a couple of reasons; first for me you be feels less of a conclusion, and has more room for possibility than you are. It also states a framework of the present instead of something that has been created by the past. I also use it as a pattern interrupt. A chance to shake the reader, you, into the present instead of just glancing through this reading mindlessly.) Is it possible that the choices made that have put you here are not yours and you are actually not living your own life? Please check out Jon Gabriel and the Gabriel Method for more on this idea.[V]

What if suffering is just a choice, and you can choose not to suffer?

Pain may be an inevitability of life, or maybe situations that are uncomfortable are part of life, but suffering is a choice. You can choose to suffer the effects of a situation or event that happens to you. You can choose how long you would like to suffer. It is your choice. Society may show you that the right thing to do is to suffer for a long period after a death, divorce, or other loss, but really it is up to you how long, or how deeply — or at all you require to suffer. How can you choose not to suffer?

How would you like to view the event? Is it just part of your life? Or do you let it stop your life and take over, forever or for awhile, altering the course you are on?

If we choose to wallow in the mire of suffering with an event that has happened in our lives, does it not effectively put the rest of one's life on hold?

It can be quite like the toppling of dominoes. By paying our attention to the loss in the past, do we miss the awareness of what is possible in the now? And what other dominoes of our lives will fall due to that lack of awareness?

What if you looked at the painful or uncomfortable events of your life as just an event or part of the experience – as something from which to learn, to grow?

One of the best tools I have developed to break me of this habit of staying with a past experience, of wallowing in the sorrow of it, is to pose this question: To whom does this belong?

You can ask yourself this question when you find yourself living in your head with the thoughts of loss, or any thoughts that prevent you from being in the present.

Just simply ask, to whom does this though belong – me or someone else? If simply asking the question gives you a feeling of being lighter, it is someone else's thought. No worries on who it belongs to, just say, "Return that thought to sender with consciousness." If you get that these thoughts belong to you, just ask this instead: "How does it get any better than this? Or ask "What else is possible?"

Keep asking these questions, or "returning to sender" until you begin to feel lighter. You will find yourself being more present and available for the awareness that being in the present brings.

Your suffering will lighten with it.

What if there is no blame?

Howard Jones wrote about this in the 1980's with the song "No One Ever is to Blame." So what if he had awareness about this? What would we have if there was no blame?[VI]

At first blush this statement may sound as a way to brush off responsibility (yikes, that is a heavy word), but I'll show you how it can work in a different way. What if we looked at everything we do, or others do, as just a choice – a choice made with all the awareness (or not) available at the time? If we disempower the choice by assigning blame, we remove the power of remaining in the question because we have just concluded that the only possibility here is that we, or others, are at fault. What else is possible after that? Is

there any new growth or new choice possible, or do we now lock ourselves into the story that the choice of laying blame has created?

Of course, you can always choose yourself out of this story, or out of any story, at any time. That is the point here. Another thought for you here is the "wrongness of me" thing that so many of us do. By accepting blame for a choice that we made, what kind of effect does that then have on us? What story will that lock us into and how will it define the place we continue to create from? Does that now create a story of us not being worthy of great things in our lives because we suck? What does that energy attract to us other than more events to fulfill the story of unworthiness?

On a side note, what effect can that have on the body? How many of you reach to food or sugar-laden beverages to soothe that feeling of not being worthy?

This is not to suggest that there is anything wrong with those choices of food or drink, but to just be aware of those choices when you make them– and to be aware of what they are contributing to your life and your body. With consciousness of our choices comes the awareness of what they are contributing to us, and then comes the ability to choose differently when those choices no longer suit us.

So what if you applied consciousness to the choice to attach blame?

Who are you trying to please?

A Parent? Teacher? Lover? Sibling? Society? What power are we giving away when we try to please someone else?

I have had countless clients over the years that were in the gym with me because someone else was putting pressure on them to lose weight and get into shape. Some of this is programming that goes back years or even decades! A father, mother, teacher or coach had called them fat, or put them on an unnecessary diet, so these clients have walked around all these years believing that they weren't good enough because they weren't the "perfect" size! Never mind the fact that all of us are different.

You may not fit into a size 0, but do you really have to? Could you really, given that you are built differently than the "ideal" person? So, what if you are constantly trying to please someone either currently or from your past? What happens if you "fail" at achieving that person's goal for you? What food looks good for you at that moment?

Is there a cycle that is created by this? I can't achieve what _____ (enter any name here) would like of me to be perfect, so I'll just have some more _____ (enter any favorite food that helps soothe the emotional pain).

You know, you are not wrong for doing this. The food doesn't require anything from you, and it fills the hole that is left from that other person not loving you just the way you are. But is there really a hole there? Are you really ever going to be filled up by someone else's love by becoming some ideal that they have formed for you in their own head?

Let me ask you something: If someone told you what to eat and not to eat, would you be inclined to defy them and do what you want to do- to eat what you want to eat? Would you still eat the taboo foods because they are far more exciting at that point?

And what else would be possible if you were not trying to please someone else, or trying to look like or act like what this person sees as perfect? What would you actually choose for yourself?

This goes for both the societal pressure to look a certain way and to eat a certain way. What would you choose for yourself without having to be what society deems as "attractive?" Ask yourself these questions and sense and see what awareness comes up for you.

What if you followed that awareness?

What if you let go of your or anyone else's need to be right?

How much of a burden is having to always be right? Right for everyone else to prove that you are worthy, better than, or at least equal to everyone else around you? You have the best answer, the best way to do everything. How heavy is that?

Are you done carrying the weight of that?

It is as simple as this: you have your way of doing things, I have mine, and other people have theirs. What if being right only applies to what is right for you? And what if what we perceive as right for us is determined by us, only us, and our awareness?

What if you just stopped worrying about how everyone else thinks or does things, and instead you just focused on you? How much of the weight you are carrying is locked up in carrying the burden of everyone else's choices?

What would happen if you just set that s#*& down, and let everyone else make choices that work for them?

And on the flip side, what if you stopped accepting what everyone else says is right for you and just did what you know is right for you?

This is your choice.

The power is in the question

Answers. It is always about answers with humans.

Since the dawn of our reality here we've sought out the answers to the questions about why we are here and what we are doing. I've had this thought for some time now – that we as humans have a need to qualify and quantify everything. That somehow by doing this we now know where and what it all is.

But what if that is all a lie?

What if all the qualification and quantification, the conclusions and judgments and the labels are just limitations, just enough to keep us rooted here in this reality? Just enough to make it all seem somewhat more believable?

The answers give us all reference points to help us feel more stable or safer. Stepping out of this place, this comfort zone of answers, is scary. It has caused more than its share of hyperventilation, sweating, and shaking. But what has happened every time someone has braved this boundary to ask more questions and to see what lies beyond– to see what else is possible? We as a society have moved forward. Is there something special about the people who create new and life-changing stuff?

Is there something that they have that the rest of us somehow don't?

No.

They just never stopped asking questions about what else is possible.

As a body builder I kept asking questions. I see now that it is just a natural process when we get ourselves involved in something that gives us bliss. We naturally want to get better at what we are doing. So we keep asking questions about it and applying the awareness that we receive in the answers.

We constantly evolve, grow, and get better at what we do. I believe the question lies at the heart of creation.

An answer or conclusion does not continue to create. It stays in its judgment, never to be more than that, never to become the butterfly of creation it can be. When you think about the creation process involved in something that gives you great bliss, ask the question:

Why not use this same process on my life as a whole?

Why wouldn't we use the same questioning process on our lives? Aren't our lives blissful?

Your life is not blissful?

Then why not start with questioning that?

See how powerful you are with the questions?

What if you looked at your life from
a point of view of abundance?

The programming of not enough is all around us. It is purely our construct, though.

It is completely our choice to be in lack. Is this feeling of not enough creating this "grab everything we can" attitude?

Is this feeling of not enough creating the need to fill ourselves with food to fill an imaginary hole that that sense of lack created?

What if everything you have, everyone you have in your life, right now is fulfilling?

Would that be enough for you? Isn't your life exactly how you have lined things up for yourself at this precise moment in time?

What if you came at your day with the thought of "My life is exactly how I have lined things up for myself at this precise moment in time"?

What changes for you when you think that you have it all? Peace? Calm? Does it feel light to think about having abundance right now?

Would that be a sign to you that you do indeed have abundance? That everything in the universe is yours? That you are connected to it and part of it all?

How do you reach this space every day?

Try having gratitude for everything in your life right now. Just stop every once in awhile and be thankful for the gift that your life is. You can thank the universe for what it is that you would desire in your life as well, just as if you already have it– because you do! No matter how small they seem, be thankful for all of the experiences in your life.

That is all that this life is, a collection of experiences. You can shape these experiences however you choose. If you choose to live in the abundance of life, that is what there is for you. If you choose to live in the lack of life, then that is what is there for you.

It is all your choice!

If you look at your life from a point of view of abundance, what shifts for you?

So much of our lives are based on lack– not enough money, not enough food, not enough time, not enough love. But this is what drives us to work harder, you say– to get up and go to our jobs, to fight traffic, deal with customers, clients, and patients just to be able to bring home more. We never quite have enough, so we have to go back to work tomorrow.

But what if all that you have right now, in this moment, is all that you need? What if everything that you need is right there for you? What is all that is required is that you ask for it? What if there is no such thing as lack or not enough?

What would your life be like to just know that everything that you will ever require to not only survive but to thrive is there?

Let's take the issue of not enough love and look at it closely.

What if you loved yourself?

What if you were the only person in the world?

What if you were the only one experiencing this life, this reality right now?

What would you do with yourself?

How would you really think about yourself?

Another question for you: Those thoughts you have of not loving yourself- are they yours or someone else's?

When you ask yourself that question, do you feel lighter? Chances are the thoughts belong to someone else. Being the amazing psychic antenna that you are, you picked up on someone else's unloving thoughts. From where do these thoughts originate?

Is it possible that by seeing the best of everyone, and by measuring ourselves at our worst against that, we create a sense of not being worthy of being loved?

What if there was no competition to be in with anyone?

What if you create your world and your relationship with yourself from the point of view that no one can be you better that you can? And you can't be anyone else better than they can be themselves?

See if that can shift the competition and unworthiness out of your thoughts.

Be you. Honor you. Love you!

What do you know about yourself, that
you are not telling yourself?

Are you in the wrong job, wrong relationship, wrong house, or wrong town for you?

And are you just sucking it up because that is just the way it is? Have you forgotten who you are? Have you forgotten what you really desire to do?

So many of us stuff those feelings so far down inside that we forget about them altogether. Sometimes we just don't acknowledge those feelings at all. We just don't tell ourselves what they are.

What if that bit of knowledge about you is creating the dis-ease or weight gain with which you are currently dealing?

Right now, I have a question for you: If money, time, the people you are with, where you live, or what job you have weren't issues, what would you do?

Right there! That thought you had right before you shoved it back down deep inside in the hole of no possibility? Pull it back out! Is it really a truth for you?

No matter how far away from "reality" it may seem, what if you explored that thought?

Does the thought of that excite you? Does it give you a sense of bliss when you indulge the fantasy?

What if you followed it for real?

Don't just write it off as impossible, because the only limitation here is your thoughts.

Just saying! Do you suppose your dis-ease or weight gain has anything to do with you living an unauthentic you?

Just let go!

Let go of what, you ask.

What would happen if you let go of your "story?" What do you have left of you? What do you have available for you?

Can you move forward into a new chapter of your life while still hanging onto the old one?

It's kind of like reading a book: How can you really dive into a new chapter or page if you are still trying to digest the last one?

Trust yourself. Trust the universe. It has your back!

How much of your relationship with food doesn't even belong to you?

For so many of us our parents are the source for everything we learn at a young age. They teach us everything by modeling, mostly in the way they act and how they do things. This can also be mirrored in the relationship we have with our bodies and with food. What did you eat growing up? How did you eat it?

Most likely, your parents and upbringing is what structured how and what you choose to eat.

Think about this: How did your mother and father think about the food they ate? Was there a conscious or unconscious choice? Did either of them have judgment about types of food at all? Did you learn this as well?

Guess what? Just because your parents, or anyone else, has this particular relationship with food does not mean you have to as well! Your relationship with food is determined by one thing: You.

What if you direct your relationship with food based upon your own thoughts?

I have an experiment for you:

What if the next 3 days you practice gratitude for your body? Start by picking statements like "Thank you, body, for this experience of life," or "Thank you, body, for all that you do for me daily, and "Thank your body for the communication you give me about what works and doesn't work for you."

See if you can work your way into thanking it for being so wonderful and beautiful!

Take note of how your food choices do or don't shift. This may take more than three days, and it may take less time. But what if you treated your body with kindness, and then it started asking for more kindness in the form of food choices?

What if you thought about food differently?

What do you know about the food choices you make that no one else knows but you?

You've been told by "them" that this food or that food will cause you to get fat. What if that is just a story and you can instead write your own story about food?

Back to the question of what do you know about it:

Our bodies all want something different and at different times. They are pretty specific about what they require and when they require it. What if we shut off our knowing of that in favor of the story someone else is telling about food — about what will work and when?

Sure, the diets that others create can and do work, but if that diet or way of eating isn't yours, isn't a way of eating that is a truth to you, will it ever work?

And if it does, will it work for the rest of your life?

For the most part the fitness industry operates on a deprivation mode. Take these foods out of your diet and never, ever eat them again or you will get fat! How does that story feel to you?

Light or heavy?

I can only assume that what most of you got while reading this was a heavy feeling. It maybe just mine, so check in with yourself. Don't just buy my story! Deprivation diets feel heavy to me because they are just not sustainable. If you completely remove something from your diet, never to eat it again, what kind of energy does that create?

Does it remove any other possibility for you? Does it remove the possibility of that food ever being a contribution to you? What if moderation in how we eat is a contribution?

We are trained in this society to eat and to eat a lot! One of the ways we express love for each other is through food. Providing food for someone is a basic desire, left over from times when finding food was a way of life. So when we found it, we provided for everyone and feasted!

That may work for our bodies once in a while, and as a matter of fact studies have shown that this is one of the ways our bodies respond to a diet and lose weight. It is a form of the paleo diet that is gaining popularity right now, and it used to be called the caveman diet. This diet alternated daily periods of fasting and a big feast at night.

We feast all the time, with breakfast, lunch, and dinner, and with snacks in between and after dinner. What if that desire to feast all the time is contributing to being overweight?

What could you choose differently?

I've made mention of this here, but what if it is the judgment we have of the food that is creating the environment for the body to store the calories as fat?

If you think it will make you fat, and you hold guilt about eating it, what energy does that send to your body? To the universe?

What, then, will possibly show up for you?

What if you looked at food and eating from a point of view of balance instead of deprivation?

Are you eating because you are hungry, or just because?

Sometimes our bodies don't require food as an energy source. There are unlimited possibilities of energy for us and our bodies in the universe!

What if you just asked you body if it requires food, water, or energy in another form?

Try it next time you think you are hungry, and see what awareness pops for you.

What fixed points of view about your body can you go monkey ninja on?

What don't you like about your body?

Have you decided that it will never change?

Have you locked into being so by deciding that it will never change?

Never get better?

What if in creating the conclusions of what you don't like about your body, or that those things will never change, locks those stories into being? Now your body is not able to show up as anything else — like the change you really desire?

What if you thought of the story as only a temporary one — one that you can change by choosing something different? By choosing to look at your body as an amazing physical manifestation for you?

What do I mean by going monkey ninja on that point of view? Destroy it. Let go of it. Put it down. Return it to where it came from. What if you got radical on your fixed points of view by destroying them and asking what else is possible here?

Keep asking that. Listen for the awareness that comes and follow what feels light for you. The new awareness might guide you to the body that you desire, but you wouldn't want that. That might be too much joy!

If you let go of the definitions of yourself,
would you find yourself lighter?

This question kind of goes along with having fixed points of view, since our definitions are fixed points of view, but what I would like to look at is how we define ourselves by our jobs, our relationships, our hobbies, our stuff (houses, cars, clothes, trips, money we have or don't have), and of course, what we look like.

Another thing to consider are the labels we put on ourselves, including straight or gay, introvert or extrovert, the color of our skin, where we are from, our religion, our age, gender, and on and on. What if by setting those definitions of who we are, we limit our possibilities and create a dis-ease in our bodies?

You are an infinite being, with infinite possibilities for your experience here in this human form. What if defining who you are actually creates a limit that in turn creates a stress that your body responds to by creating a dis-ease, or by storing fat, or creating pain, or any other possible dis-ease or un-joy? What if you just choose to be who you be without the limits of definition? How does that feel?

Would your body respond by letting go of the pain, dis-ease, and weight?

I can tell you that when I choose to be who I am, choose to be in the moment instead of defining myself by mistakes of the past or concerns for the future, and when I drop the definitions of man, father, or trainer, my aches and pains disappear. I also notice I don't crave certain foods to soothe my bruised ego or my shattered emotions.

I just am…Happy!

Try it, or not. Your choice, as always!

What if the key to your weight loss lies in honoring yourself?

What does it mean to honor yourself?

The fitness and weight loss industry has traditionally used judgment, denial, and even borderline abuse to generate its revenue, asking that in exchange for the weight that you will lose, you must completely give up the foods you like to eat and do these workouts several times a week. Some of them are pretty brutal workouts, especially for someone who has never worked out before. I know. I used to offer that as my business model. Sometimes, given the chance, a trainer will grow from that experience and begin creating programs that are tailored for the client. These are designed to bring them along at a pace that is not so fast as to be an abuse, but not to slow as to be a waste of money and time.

So what if honoring yourself and your body were keys to your weight loss?

What if that bootcamp class that your friends are raving about, but you have questions about doing, isn't the right choice for you?

What if the latest, greatest, end-all diet that is working for "millions" isn't the right one for you?

So by doing those plans, even when they don't feel right, are you dishonoring you?

What if you instead did the movement/exercise and meal planning that you and your body find blissful?

Having said this, doing or changing nothing in your plan will most likely keep you where you currently are. So always knowing that you have a choice in this, what if you choose to move and to choose foods that are nurturing to your body?

How do you do this?

What if you followed what felt light?

Seek out awareness that will help guide you with this, of course. So with the infinite number of choices that you have, ask questions and follow your awareness. You really can't make a wrong choice because you always have the choice to choose again!

Would that feel like an honoring of you and your body?

What if the "facts" or "reality" change depending on how you look at them?

So what would happen if you looked at the "problem" of weight loss differently?

Do the "facts" or "reality" of how you got that way and how you are supposed to "fix" it change?

If you saw the weight gain as a way for your body to try and tell you something, would you change how you felt about weight gain?

Would weight gain become a communication from your body instead of a betrayal?

And if it was just a simple communication, would your body then respond to your questions of how to let go of the weight?

Think about how you like to be treated by others. If you are treated as an adversary, are you more or less likely to respond to the requests of the person or people asking you to do something? What happens when you are treated with kindness?

What if you treated and asked your body with kindness, and saw what your body was doing as a kindness as well?

Does the "reality" of your situation change? If it doesn't for you, what questions could you ask that would change your "reality"?

You are the miracle

Have you ever even considered that — that you just being you is the miracle?

How does it feel to hear that? To say, "I am the miracle!" to yourself, or even out loud? Try it and see what shifts. Does it make you feel uncomfortable to even think it?

Have you for so long been beating yourself up for not being worthy that even thinking about you being a miracle doesn't feel right?

Here is one place where I would urge you to step into the uncomfortable and say it to yourself over and over – because you are the miracle! Now, just get out there and be the miracle.

Be you!

Get Uncomfortable

It's interesting that this one landed here, so many pages into the book. I find this to be the greatest contribution to my overall bliss!

Every time I do something that is uncomfortable for me, like going to a large group meeting and talking with people, or when I started shooting videos and putting them out there on YouTube and Facebook for public consumption and judgment, or just riding my bike passed a point that I thought I could go, I find amazing things about myself, and about life, that I would never have experienced had I stayed comfortable.

See what you think!

So you may be comfortable now. Even with the weight you would like to lose, there is a routine, some habits that you do that are just part of your day. Well, that routine got you what you got. Are you going to stay with it and expect anything to change? Hmmm…

What if you got out there and challenged yourself – challenged yourself to make different food choices than you do now?

What if you challenged yourself to actually get that exercise that you have been threatening, promising yourself that you would do?

This is what I mean by get uncomfortable. Some call it "stepping outside your comfort zone." What will you find there? Only you can know what that is by experiencing it. I can tell you it will be different than what you have experienced to this point.

You may find hidden talents or desires. It may suck or it may be fun as hell!

I can promise to you that it will be different. It will stretch you as a person, and it will be a contribution to your target of weight loss. Every little thing you do from gaining consciousness around what you eat, to the movements and exercise you choose to do, will contribute to the overall target of weight loss. Toss in some reprogramming of the thought loop running through your head from some form of "I Suck" to the probably uncomfortable now, "I am Awesome" will be a contribution as well.

Wrap all that up into one new uncomfortable routine or habit, and you have a clear path to your target.

Chapter Two

Your Body

What would it take to feel proud, confident, and super sexy, not to mention light, easy, and fun in and with your body now? Love and allowance for what your body is now will open the path of communication between you two, giving the best chance for the awareness needed to get your body where you would like it to be – and how to get there.

What is that Extra Weight anyway?

What if the extra weight you have put on has nothing to do with the food you eat, or the type of exercise you do or don't do? What if it is all just your body's response to the judgments that are heaped onto it? Judgments from you, judgments from others, the stories you have bought into about how your life should go, how you should look, the things you should be doing. And what if all the while you are ignoring who it is that you be?

Just imagine the internal conflict of that. What are the possibilities that this could create? Dis-ease? Obesity? Depression?

Now imagine the possibilities of filling that space with something. Food?

And imagine that the food will never quite satisfy that kind of hunger, but it's all you know to do. So, more food, more food, more food, and yet you never quite feel fulfilled. Then your body steps in and creates an environment to support that, by slowing down your metabolism, creating cravings for certain foods, and storing fat. It cycles around.

You do have choices here.

What if you stepped into being you and started doing the things that you have always had thoughts of doing, but pushed aside in favor of another path. Maybe that path wasn't even yours! You try to fill that emptiness with food, instead of what you and your body are craving.

What are the possibilities with you and your body when you choose for you?

What if it is not about perfect?

What if life is not about the perfect body, the perfect life, the perfect spouse, or the perfect job? What is that? Do the definitions of perfect even belong to you, or are you doing this life to keep up with someone else?

Are you doing this life just to look good in someone else's eyes, or to fit in with a certain group of people? What if you have the perfect life—right now, in this very moment, but you are more concerned with what you didn't do, what you should do, what you look like, how your clothes fit, or if they are the right clothes in the first place?

And by focusing your attention on these thoughts and concerns, you missed the moment and its perfection. Take a deep breath. Feel it enter your lungs. Take a really deep belly breath. Feel your feet on the ground. Feel the wind or sunshine if you are outside. Listen to your surroundings. What do you hear?

What if every moment if perfectly set up just for you, if you are only available to enjoy it? What if your body is perfect the way it is right now given what it is trying to do for you?

What is your body telling you?

Have you ever listened to your body and what it would like to eat, drink, or do based on the thoughts you are sending it of what a perfect body should look and feel like? Did you follow through with what your body's requested, or did you force your body to do something or eat something because it was what you are "supposed to do"?

Your body knows what to do. All that's required is that you listen to its awareness and requests when you tell it what it is you would desire. If you tell it that it is betraying you or that it is fat, or it sucks or is no good, what do you think it will respond with?

Is it possible that your body will listen to what you tell it and respond with signals to create and to match those thoughts for you?

What else is possible if you listen to the signals your body is giving you? You know, the signals that tell you to stop eating, or to refrain from that exercise today, or just to slow down?

You can learn from the signals your body gives you about food. If, for example, there is a food that you eat that consistently causes you to bloat and gain a few pounds the next day, listen to your body and limit (or eliminate) that food from your diet. You may be surprised at the effect down the road. Taking the time to listen to your body can have amazing results with your overall health.

So, what if you listened to your body? After all, it is your primary life partner.

What if you have allowance for you and your body now?

What would it feel like to never judge your body unkindly again? What would it feel like to never look in the mirror and see a "fat" person staring back?

What I would like you to realize is that the term "fat" is just a label, a judgment. Something else to consider this: Is the term "fat" even a useful adjective? After all, you may have hair on your head, but we don't call you hair, do we?

If you look at it, we have at this point in societal history made having "excess" fat an undesirable thing. But there have been periods in our history when this wasn't the case. Fat has over time been accepted and even considered attractive. And come to think of it, how many of us might consider someone who carried extra fat on their body attractive now, if it weren't for the collective "brain?" Beauty is in the eye of the beholder.

Some of us are attracted to thinner, some thicker. And sometimes the thought in our head about what and who we are attracted to isn't our thought at all. Sometimes we will see someone that isn't our "type" and find them attractive, but we walk right on past a possibility of a great relationship because that person isn't our "type." What am I getting at with all of this?

I'm getting to the point of allowance for our bodies the way they are. Part of the attraction we have for each other is that confidence we have in ourselves. That knowing that we are the best at being who we are, no matter what size we are. With that comes a knowing that the "right" person will be there. Chasing an ideal built on our size, or how we look to become attractive to someone else, is just fake. And a relationship built on fake will never work.

The other part of this is an awareness of your body is doing just what you are asking of it to do. Now, this isn't said to provoke you to go into a wrongness of you, just to give you some awareness of how your body works, so maybe you can find some gratitude for it. First and foremost, our bodies are designed to keep us alive, so the functions of the body run to do just that. Having said that, what if…

What if your body wants to put on fat any time it decides that storing fat is the best way to keep you safe?

Oh great. My body is working against me!

Well, what if it isn't? What if all of the daily stress, added up over time, has created the signal to your body that putting on fat is the best way to keep you safe?

I'm talking about stresses like, work, kids, paying bills, the judgments on you from others, from yourself, your past that you still live in, the future that you're stressed about, and so on. What if all of that has told your body that it's time to store fat?

This isn't my idea, but it rings of a truth with me given the nature of what I have seen and heard over the years of training people. Jon Gabriel has created the Gabriel Method based on this very concept.[VII] The difference between people who store excess fat and people who don't is just as simple as people who store extra fat just have their fat-storing mechanism turned on. There is nothing wrong with you. Your body is just trying to protect you.

Let me shuffle back a bit here and tell you something you may or may not know: Being fat is not a problem to be solved. It is a symptom of another action. Our bodies store fat due to something else that is happening within us, physically, emotionally or mentally. Our bodies will protect us from harm and dying. And one of the ways it will do this is to shift the hormonal signals of the body to slow down metabolism and crave certain foods in order to store fat. The body may perceive the "threat" as a need to survive a famine, or drop in ambient temperature and trigger the fat-storing mechanisms. But just addressing the physical part of this via diet and exercise does not always solve the issue. Most of the time a body will revert back to its fat storing state. Why?

It's simply because the source issue remains, and the body still gets the signal to protect you and just put the fat back on. Most likely the stressor in your life, which your body interpreted as a need to store fat, is still around, and still not being addressed.

Our bodies are still designed like our ancestors' bodies, when our main concerns were when we would eat again, how we would stay warm when out in the cold, and how we could keep from getting eaten ourselves! In the first two instances, a prolonged famine or cold temperatures, the body's response is to store fat, for protection from famine (because fat is a great source of calories) and from cold temperatures (because being a little bigger protects you and your organs from freezing). In the second instance of actually being threatened as the prey of something else, we drop the body fat to become quicker so that we might flee and survive.

So how about some stress relieving techniques during your day? How about 30 to 60 minutes of exercise as an amazing stress reducer? Or consider some quiet time to reflect or meditate. How about shutting off the TV an hour before bed to read something light or uplifting? How about playing with your kids or pets? Maybe make love to your partner?

Do you think you might fit some of these into your day and then see what shifts for you?

In chapter 4 of this book you'll find a list of common life stressors that my clients have

brought up to me many times. With that list I have some questions you can ask, and some ways to reframe your thoughts around those stressors. I also pose a list of things that bring joy and bliss just to jog your mind a bit about what you may already have in your world that are wonderful.

*What if your weight gain has nothing
to do with the food you eat?*

But isn't the weight I have put on a direct result of the calories I ingest? It depends.

What if your food choices have nothing to do with you being undisciplined? Hear me out here. What if your food choices are driven by something else?

So our thoughts go, so our body goes. What if the thoughts you have running on a loop in your subconscious actually are giving your body the signal to store fat, creating the cravings and desires for foods and amounts of foods that you normally wouldn't choose? And what if your body is doing all of this in an effort to protect you?

So is it really about the food? You could change the way you are eating, lose some weight, and never really address the thoughts in your subconscious mind — thus you'll find yourself reaching for the same foods again, only to put the weight back on that you lost. Does this sound familiar?

So what if instead of dealing with a symptom as a problem to solve, we sought the source. What if we seek out the reason a body puts the weight on in the first place? What if we reprogram your subconscious with a new loop?

It's like when you learn a new task, job, or hobby like playing a musical instrument. At first you are very conscious of every step you take in learning the new task, but after some repetition, you find yourself doing it second nature. What if your subconscious thoughts are the same? What if the ones you have going on now are attracting exactly what you are asking for? What if you consciously reprogrammed them with a new "loop" — one that supports what you desire now?

What if you replaced the thoughts you have in your head of "I am not good enough, I will never lose this fat, I am fat, I am unlovable, I am not worthy," with new ones? You could do this in the morning by saying things to yourself like, "I am amazing," "I am infinitely lovable," or, "My body is awesome!"

Feel free to use anything that comes to your awareness. Repeat it throughout the day when you remember. A good time to say them is when you find yourself thinking of the other, non-supportive thoughts.

What if you stopped comparing yourself to others?

What if you strived to be the best you that you can be? The chances of you being someone else are pretty slim, so what else do you have? So, why would you compare yourself to someone else? Wouldn't that just set you up for disappointment? If you expect to be like someone else and then fall short, what does that do for you? What does it do for your sense of self worth? What if you realized and reveled in the wonderment that is you?

You – the amazing, wonderful, magical you!

Can anyone else ever be who you be with the same magic that you bring to being you? Can you really compare yourself to anyone else? Really? It's the proverbial comparing apples to oranges. It can't be done. They are different. You can like one or the other, or both, but comparing them to each other really can't be done.

One other thought here: So often we are looking at someone at their best and comparing that to what we see as our worst. When we are out in public, most often we are looking and acting our best. Most of the time we are hiding all of our insecurities underneath that well-thought out and put together exterior, just hoping that they won't be discovered. All of this primping and effort just to keep us from being undesirable and left out of all the cool kid games.

This is fine; it is an interesting point of view. But next time you find yourself saying, "So-and-so has it all together, I wish I could be more like her or him," remember that they are probably thinking the same thing about you.

Yup! They are...

If you were the only person around, who would you judge your body and yourself against?

Think about this. You are it. You are the only person in the world.

Would you have any use to judge your body in and unkind manner? Would you really call yourself fat or ugly? How about unworthy or unlovable?

Who would be there for you to compare yourself to or to be in competition with? Who would be there to do the reality show with?

What if you treated your body with kindness — in everything that you say to it and about it — and in everything you do to it and with it?

What would that feel like for you?

If you think about it, you are the only one you can be. You can't be your friends, your family, or the hot actress on TV. Those people are already taken. So why compare yourself to them and beat yourself up over not being them? Is that a kindness to you?

Mind you, this is not to make yourself wrong for choosing to do that, just to let you know you have a choice here. Choose to be you regardless of what friends, family, or society say about it, or choose to try to fit into the narrow mold that is presented to us as acceptable.

What choice feels lighter for you?

Your body knows what to do with real food!

Processed food, fast food, genetically modified organisms (GMO's), imitation sugars, hydrogenated/ partially hydrogenated oils, imitation colors/ fragrances, flavor enhancers, preservatives– what do they all have in common?

They are mostly man-made and manipulated food-like substances. What does this mean to you and your body?

Our bodies haven't yet evolved to using these new substances, substances that can trick our bodies into signaling functions that aren't intended (and that include weight gain, inflammation, and cancer cell growth).

So what is happening here? Fake foods and processed or fast foods are for the most part designed to get you to eat more! Why? To keep you buying more of them, of course! To create the need to eat more, the companies that create these "foods" make more money. It's as simple as that!

The chronic consumption of these "food" and the inflammation that they can cause are creating the health issues we see popping up at an alarming rate.

Know this: Our bodies just know what to do with real, whole, organic foods, and that includes foods like real sugar (not processed table sugar), pasture butter, and whole eggs. It can and does use these foods appropriately. It can and does shut off the need to keep eating these foods.

So what to do here? Have the awareness that this is possibly happening when you choose to eat processed foods, and as best as you can, and as often as you can, choose whole organic foods to eat instead. This will go a long way to preserving and enhancing your physical and mental health!

Chronic Inflammation: What is it?

We are all aware of inflammation—the swelling that happens when we injure ourselves, right? That would be acute inflammation. It usually is easy to deal with and required by the body to heal whatever is going on. Chronic inflammation happens when we continually assault the body and injure it over and over again. It creates a state in which our bodies are always inflamed somewhere, or in multiple places. What can cause chronic inflammation?

Simply what we choose to put into or onto our bodies, usually over and over again, can cause chronic inflammation. Sugar, processed foods, chemical ingredients, alcohol, cigarettes, drugs—anything that we do to excess, day after day, can cause chronic inflammation. It can even be something that we have been told is "healthy" for us.

Your trainer or nutritionist, or that great diet plan that is guaranteed not to fail, may be causing or contributing to the chronic inflammation. For example: Did you know that oatmeal, Greek yogurt, and salmon are inflammatory for about 85 percent of the population?[VIII] And these are staples of the weight loss industry.

Foods that cause inflammation:

So inflammation happens in our bodies for a variety of reasons. The ones with which we are most familiar are the inflammation that appears after a cut or bruise. Blood rushes to the area, bringing the stuff necessary to heal that wound, but what about other inflammations?

We can pretty much have inflammations throughout or bodies. Things like arthritis, colitis, hepatitis-- anything with an "itis" after it is an inflammation.

But what is it?

Inflammation is the body's attempt at self-protection, its aim being to remove harmful stimuli, including damaged cells, irritants, or pathogens and then to begin the healing process.

So what if foods can cause inflammation? Yes, food! You didn't think about that one, did you? What if that food that you constantly eat is causing chronic inflammation, creating a state in which your body never fully heals from the harmful stimuli?

The result could be that you have a situation where other processes of your body are impaired, or stop working all together. Digestion is one.

If the foods you are eating cause an irritation in your digestive tract, leading to chronic inflammation, irritable bowel syndrome, Crohn's disease, or colitis, your digestion will be impaired and nutrients from other foods you eat won't be properly absorbed, which leads to other malnutrition issues. Yeah, I said malnutrition.

Haven't thought about that while living in a modern society, huh? With all the food available to you at any given notice, you could be malnourished?

It has been suggested that all of the diseases we suffer from stem from inflammation.

Hmmm... What else is possible here?

What if you had an awareness of the foods that cause you issues? What would you do then as a kindness to your body? Would you continue to eat them or switch to something else? Could you ask questions of your body about what foods it would require? How about questions about ease around the foods you are eating?

Again, there are some really common foods that cause inflammation for a majority of the population. These include some fitness and nutrition industry standards that I mentioned earlier, like oatmeal, Greek yogurt, and salmon. Check in with yourself and see if any of these feel like they are causing you problems, since they absolutely do for many. And note that you certainly may be in the 15 percent with no problems at all here.

See what happens when you ask questions, and check out the book *The Plan* by Lyn Genet to find out more about this. Good book![IX]

Are you choosing to fill a hole with food?

What is missing in your life? The perfect love? The perfect job? The perfect life in general?

Have you not defined what it is that is missing? You just know something is missing?

Good.

Leave it free of definition right now, and I am going to ask you to explore something with me. What if what is missing is your love and kindness for you?

What did that just stir up for you?

Don't push it away! Don't bury those feelings. Those may be creating a "black hole" for you, a hole to be filled by other things in life — things like houses, cars, clothes, shoes, trips, people, drugs, alcohol, and food. But in the nature of it being a "black hole," it has an insatiable appetite! More, more, more! (Did anyone else start pumping their fist and singing Billy Idol right there?)

Back to the feelings that came up for you. Unworthy of love? Was that one of them? Or at least some variation on that theme, like too fat, too ugly, too boring, too whatever to be truly loved by anyone, so why should I love myself?

Yeah.

To whom does that belong to anyway– you, or someone else?

If you just got a lighter feeling with that question, would you be willing to let go of that and return it to sender (whomever it belongs to) with consciousness?

Don't worry, you can't create a bigger load for that person; they already have that thought. Returning the thought won't add anymore to theirs. Besides, sending it back with consciousness attached may give that person the opportunity to let go of it as well.

But if this creates some issues for you, send the energy of the thought to the Earth instead.

If you didn't get light, and the thoughts belong to you, would you be willing to let go of them? Destroy and un-create them? Once again, this all comes down to a choice. You have the choice to own these thoughts and use them or be used by them. What if we brought this back to gratitude for you and your body?

Is it the food that is making you fat, or the judgment of the food making you fat?

This may be the question that started this whole book journey for me. It was one of the first ones that I became aware of when I started asking what else is possible around food, exercise, and our relationships with our bodies. Our thoughts are creating everything around us. Everything in our lives shows up in direct relationship to our thoughts about them. Our thoughts are our filters. So is it possible that how we think about our food and the effect it has on our bodies creates the situations we experience? In other words, if you think that this or that food will make you fat, will it? Would you ask yourself if those thoughts belong to you, or to someone else?

We have so many thoughts about what food will and won't do for us in our society. It's a wonder we can eat anything and not get fat! You have that friend who can eat pretty much anything she wants, right? You always wrote that off to good genetics, right?

What if she has no judgment, no point of view about food at all? And what if she also isn't affected by anyone else's point of view?. Would you just destroy and un-create all the thoughts and judgments you have about food?

For the next three days, every time you go to eat or drink something, would you just destroy and un-create all the thoughts, feelings, judgments, and perceptions you have about that food — or that society may have about that food and you are now picking up those thoughts as your own?

See what happens with your body after doing this. Does it crave less? Do you eat less of the servings you put on the plate for yourself? What else is possible here?

Did you create a bigger body to travel in here because you bought into the idea you had to be smaller than the body you travel in?

Yeah. Interesting question, huh?

You are an infinite being. Your body is a finite one. As such, as an infinite being, you are well, infinite!

What if your body is inside you, and not the other way around? And you being the human that you are, wanting to fit into things with the rest of the humans, choose to believe the other way around? What if you stuffed your infinite being inside of this body, or at least gave it a go? But since you are infinite, you aren't fitting all that well. So, why don't we make the body bigger to accommodate? What if?

You have choice here — to expand outside of the body back into the infinite being that you are, or keep trying to be small and fit into your body. But is that a kindness to your body and you?

Just checking!

What about your body are you defending for or against?

Have you chosen that you will never have the body that you desire? That it will require too much work to get there? That you are too undisciplined to make it happen?

Lazy? Couch potato?

Are you defending for or against these points of view of your body?

"What you resist persists," said Carl Jung.[x]

Are defending for or against those points of view about your body, keeping you there? What if you let go of that right now, and know that you have choice here?

You have the choice of knowing anything is possible with your body. Just ask questions.

"Body, how would you like to lose this weight?"

What does your body tell you?

What if you did that, no matter how ridiculous or against common "sense" it seemed?

Use your awareness here. Ask questions. You know.

You know?

What if weight gain is a symptom,
not a problem to solve?

We have become so focused on the "problem" of weight and fat gain in our society. There is a multi-billion dollar a year industry created to serve this "problem," so looking at it any differently could cause substantial losses in money for a lot of businesses and people. What will this shift to a more holistic approach cause?

What if we instead viewed weight and fat gain as a sign or message from the body? What would you find out about yourself when you ask your body what it is trying to tell you?

The awareness I get is that it is something most of us are unwilling to really look at—that every thought we have, every choice we make, leads to an outcome. To look at things in your life this way is scary, but to know that you are in "charge" of it all is empowering!

Still, right now, for most of us, it is a whole lot more comfortable to think that we are not the cause of our weight gain. And when we do come to that awareness, or really most of the time it is a conclusion, we go into the wrongness of ourselves for getting ourselves overweight, and we defeat the process of weight and fat loss before it even starts.

What could your body be telling you by putting weight on? Are you not moving enough for it? Are you honoring the right movement for you? Are you feeding it too many fast foods or convenient foods and not enough of nurturing, nutritious, whole foods? Consider what are the causes of those choices.

Trust me when I say this: You are not just lazy and undisciplined! There is another thought pattern that is driving these choices for you.

What do I mean by that? Your predominant subconscious thought patterns are ruling what you attract to you and how your body is responding.

So what are those?

What if you started asking questions about and around that? And what if you began the process of reprogramming those thoughts? What if you began to visualize what it is you would like your body to be for you?

Take an honest approach to this. Ask yourself and your body what you can accomplish and what you are willing to do to get there. Listen to the awareness's that come from your body. They may show up in different ways than you are accustomed to, but most likely, you already get these messages from your body. You know the moments when you said, "I knew I shouldn't have done that!" You knew something about what you were planning to do with your body and how it would react, even before you did it. This is your body telling you what most likely will happen. Take the time to learn this language — the language that you and your body share. Your plan can and will take shape from there.

When you feel whole, do you then have the need to gain weight to try to be whole?

Unlovable. Unworthy. Not included. Less than. Not enough. Not beautiful enough. Not thin enough.

Basically any feeling of lack in your life.

Are you reaching for food, the one thing that always provides comfort for you, to fill the voids left by the feelings listed above?

When you feel worthy, how are your eating habits altered? Do you still eat the same way? Or do you find yourself reaching for different foods, or no foods at all?

What would it take for you to feel that you are worthy? To know that you are worthy?

What if you asked the question: What would it take to know that I am worthy of all the greatness that life has to offer me?

Follow the awareness's that come. No matter what that looks like, use them to step into who you be, instead of who you accept is proper for you to be. What would your life, your body, your communion with your body look like if you stepped into all of who you be? What would that attract into your life then?

I don't really like advertising slogans anymore, but this one is good: "Just Do It!"

What if you did?

> *What would happen if you stopped denying*
> *yourself and your body what you require?*

What does it feel like to think that you can have everything you require?

Again, that feeling you had the moment before you pushed it away in favor of "reality"? You know, the feeling you have right before you say to yourself that would be impossible because that is just not how my life or my reality works!

Yeah. How is that working for you? The denial of life? Of living? Of feeling alive?

You know that tight, heavy feeling you get when you have chosen against what you would like to do in favor of what you "should" do? What do you suppose that is?

What do you suppose that may be creating for you and your body?

I am not suggesting that you should just avoid all the unpleasant things in life in favor of what feels good, or just go hog wild and eat whatever you want and how much you want.

There are requirements that your body has. And there are things to do to maintain or grow your life and lifestyle.

I have a couple of tools for you here.

What if the next time you are faced with that knotted up feeling when you are about to do or eat something that doesn't feel light or right, you asked some questions around it instead of just doing it? You could ask, "Is what I am about to do a contribution to me and my body?" If you feel a "lightness," then it may be.

If it feels "heavy", but it is something that you have committed to doing for one reason or another, you could ask, "How can this task be as joyful as possible for me?"

Just listen for the awareness around it. It may just be that the time passes without you really thinking about how little fun you are having. When it comes to food, ask why you are eating it. "Will this food be a contribution to me and my body?"

If you are getting a no or a "heavy" feeling about the food you are about to eat, is there another choice? Now, ask your body what it requires: "Body, what would you like to eat, or do you require food right now?"

If you really want to eat the food in question, and you are getting a heavy feeling, you have the awareness.

Your body not only doesn't require it, it may not desire it at this time either. In knowing this, you can ask your body how you can enjoy this food with as much ease as possible.

Asking the questions and gaining awareness is the key to more consciousness in your choices, leading to more joy and ease in your life—for both you and your body. How does it get any better than that?

What did you create this body for?

Have you ever asked yourself this? Give it a try. See what awareness comes.

It may be an amazing contribution to you to know this!

It is an entrainment in our society to think that our bodies are what they are and that we have little or no control over it. Just play the hand you are dealt and that is it.

Guess what? You are only a victim of circumstance if you accept that story.

What you choose to put in, on, and around you and your body are the choices that contribute to the creation of your body!

Yeah, yeah, yeah, I hear you. The basic "blueprint" may have been there when you were born, but are you guiding the path you and your body take, or are you just letting "shit happen"?

So what did you create your body for? To sit around and watch life go by, or to jump in and create Bliss?

How could you shift your thinking to guide you and your body in a different direction? Could you do that?

What if you asked, "What else is possible with you, body?" You may be surprised!

But then again, you wouldn't want that much fun in your life!

Would ya?

*What if you could have your body look like
anything you wanted, what would it be?*

You know what? What if you just asked your body questions about how to transfer those thoughts into reality? What if it is that simple?

What if you suspended the story of "you can't do that" and asked questions instead, listening for awareness and then asking more questions?

And if living in the question is uncomfortable, what is that telling you?

Is it possible that everything that has ever been created came from a place of uncomfortable? If we remain comfortable, what does that create? Does it create?

So what if you got uncomfortable about the questions you ask in regards to your body — you know, the ones that you have been avoiding, shoved down deep inside and forgotten about? Or maybe you have never brought up those questions at all, for fear of what they may mean? Could those questions lead to creating the body you desire?

I challenge you to ask yourself this question and see what comes up: "What questions can I ask about my body right now that might change everything I thought I knew was possible with it?" Where does that lead you?

You could skip that one if you like, because it may lead to joy and THAT is definitely something you wouldn't like in your life!

Do you have Gratitude for your body?

Have you ever thanked your body for everything? How about for anything? Are you just taking for granted that it will always be there, operating just the same for you every day?

Consider what would happen if you stopped and said, "Thank you, body. Thank you for all of the experiences of life! Thank you for the smells, sights, sounds, tastes, and for everything that I touch and feel!"

On the subject of touch: What if you took time in the morning to give your body gratitude but just running your hands over your body while you thank it?

Bodies love to be touched, or haven't you noticed? Yes, you can touch yourself! LOL!

It seems as though that has become a taboo in society — to touch yourself! Are we only allowed to touch someone else? And are we only allowing someone else to touch us?

That certainly feels good too, but what would happen if you allowed yourself to show gratitude and care for YOUR body as well? Could that open up the communion with your body to have anything else be a possibility?

Would you be able to hear what your body is telling you if you just acknowledged it with gratitude? Think about how it feels when someone else acknowledges you with gratitude. Are you more open to communicating and sharing ideas with them? Would that work with your relationship with your body as well?

And while we are on the subject:

Do you have gratitude for you?

Have you thanked yourself for all that you have and continue to do and be?

What if you cut yourself some slack, my friend? What if you just acknowledge what you already know?

You are a beautiful, amazing, magical infinite being! And nothing or no one can take that away from you unless you allow it!

So what if you thanked yourself for the magic you create, you amazing being?

What if dieting is causing your body to want to be fat?

With most "diets" you are asked to remove foods from your diet. While some of these "foods," like fast foods and processed foods, are best kept to a minimum when considering a weight-loss plan, there are "diets" out there that require more drastic approaches, with complete removal of foods not just for the diet phase but possibly for the rest of your life!

Sometimes the removal of a whole food source is replaced by a proprietary laboratory creation– a "fake" food, be it a bar, a shake, or pills.

What if your body doesn't know what to do with these foods? What if in an effort to protect you from an overload of toxins rolling around through your blood stream, it does what it is designed to do—it stores the excess toxins in fat, sometimes even creating new fat cells to accommodate the overload?

If your liver is taxed by too many toxins to process, this is what your body will do to protect you.

Now another question for you, and it's a repeat of an earlier question: What if your body knows what to do with whole, real food?

If you are considering a diet that asks you to remove whole, real food from your intake, consider asking the question "Why?"

The other awareness to consider here has to do with "yoyo" dieting. Jumping from one diet, to the next, to the next can create a situation where your body will not let go of the fat.

Your body will perceive the lack of nutrients as a famine and hold onto the fat as a means of helping you survive.

If you are considering any "diet" other than just a balanced, mostly whole food approach to eating, give it a chance to work before you move on. Follow the advice that the providers of the plan are giving you. And before you start any "diet," find out if there is an exit strategy to move back into a balanced lifestyle. If it is a forever plan, ask yourself whether or not you can live the rest of your life like that. And as always, keep asking questions about the plan as you go along.

The Industrial Food Chain

The industrial food chain is full of pitfalls to be aware of, from pesticides, to herbicides, to genetically modified organisms, to the shipping, packaging, and storing of the foods. What I want to bring to light here is the method which the industrial food chain uses most often to ripen fruits and vegetables.

Usually this produce requires shipping food over fairly long distances to get to you. To ripen on the vine or tree and then ship would cause a lot of spoilage. So it's been figured out that if you put the produce in a truck filled with nitrogen, the produce will "ripen" via a fermentation method. It works, but the produce is robbed of the opportunity to fully develop and absorb as many nutrients as possible, like it would while ripening on the vine or tree.

Two things come to mind here, and one is the potential lack of nutrients compared to a fully vine or tree-ripened version. The other is the taste of the produce.

Try something here: Find a local supply of produce, something that is grown in your area. Pick a fruit or vegetable from that source. Now go to the supermarket and pick a conventional or non-organic version then do a taste test.

Another thing to consider here is the flash-frozen produce. These fruits and veggies are vine or tree-ripened and then cleaned, flash-frozen, and packaged. All the nutrients that the produce will get are in there, meaning that sometimes this may be a much more nurturing for your body.

Your best possible option in my interesting opinion is to eat as much local and organically grown food as possible, which leads me to:

Organic foods: Why?

I find it ironic that the way food has been grown for thousands of years is now called "organic" and the way food has been grown in the past maybe 100 years is called "conventional." It's seems backwards to me somehow.

But why we have organic foods — and why that choice would prove to be a contribution to your body is what I want to discuss here.

I am often asked what the difference is between organic and conventional or regular produce, meats, and grains (other than the price). Well, the industrial food industry will tell you there are no differences. Food is food. Yeah, maybe.

But consider this: The produce and grains grown either way have the potential to offer the same nutrient values, except for the produce that is picked before it's ripe and then shipped.

It's what organic does not have that has the potential to be a greater contribution to you and your body. It does not have chemical pesticides, herbicides, or fertilizers, and organic is non-genetically modified by definition – and by the rules handed down by the USDA.

With meats, animals that are deemed organic have been humanely treated throughout their life, are generally fed foods that they are intended to eat, and are not given steroids, growth hormones, or antibiotics. Usually. Sometimes an organically grown animal may be given antibiotics to protect the whole herd or flock from getting disease and dying off. Just check with the grower on this.

And the animals still may be fed something other than what they normally would eat (like corn-based feeds for cattle), as long as the corn and other ingredients were grown organically.

Want to save some confusion? When picking beef, choose 100 percent grass fed, grass-finished beef. When picking chicken, choose free-range, but find something where the birds actually are left in the yard, not just in an open pen with each other. Just ask the butcher. Whole Foods is pretty good at explaining their options.

We are also going to now start seeing genetically modified animals. There is a GMO salmon waiting approval to bring to market. What is this fish modified to do? Grow faster and subsist on a corn-based diet (salmon are carnivores by nature, so corn isn't on their diet normally and doesn't support the animal optimally).

Just an aside here, but farm-raised, corn-fed salmon is deficient in the omega-3 fatty acids that make their wild caught counterparts so potentially healthy. The pink color in wild caught salmon is there due to the large amounts of krill the salmon eat in the wild. When farm-raised salmon are fed a diet devoid of this, their meat is actually grey. The pigment is artificially added through their food to create a "normal" looking fish for consumption. These are also some of the things that can, for some, make salmon an inflammatory food.

Whew!! Enough on the salmon. Things like this are going on throughout the industry as big agri-business seeks more efficient and cost-effective ways to grow, package, ship, and store food. The awareness is that it's all about the money, not our health and well-being.

In chapter 4, I have listed foods and an easy-to-follow 4-level guide to categorize them.

Sleep. Why?

Not enough sleep is some kind of badge of honor in our society.

"I'll sleep when I am dead." How many times have you said that in your life? How long did that last before your body just said "No more," and you either got sick and had to stop and rest, or you finally fell asleep and were down for 13 hours straight?

What do you think that is?

Your body requires regular sleep.

Everyone is different—some need less and some need more, but the story here is that your body requires sleep. The body does all of its restorative work when we rest, when we sleep. It has the chance then to repair the damage to muscle, skin, bone, organs, and connective tissue while we sleep.

Our brains do a pretty cool thing to while we sleep, too. They process events and thoughts from the day, giving us the possibility of reducing or eliminating the stress brought about by them.

Restoration.

Sleep is a chance to restore our bodies and brains to a state that makes it possible to now deal with a new day in a more contributive way.

So, what are some ways to help you sleep? Well, for one, turn off the TV. As a matter of fact, remove the TV from your bedroom. Get used to the bedroom being for just that—the bed.

Next, write down your "to do" list before you sleep. This way, you can get tasks cleared from your mind and not have to roll them all around going, "I gotta remember to do that tomorrow!"

You know you do that!

Try reading something fun or inspirational before you go to sleep. Yes, put away the work and just enjoy the few minutes before you sleep. The productivity that you receive the next day because you slept will more than make up for the time.

How about just talking with a loved one, your spouse, your partner? What if you visited with him or her a bit before you slept? Novel idea, huh?

So, what if you listened to your body's request for sleep?

Chapter Three

MOVEMENT

When it comes to movement and exercise, if
it isn't fun, then why are you doing it?

What do I mean by this question? We have this entrained sense that in order for anything to be worthwhile, that it has to be work. Almost drudgery. I have seen this over and over again in the gym over the years — a lot of people, on the cardio equipment, or running through the machines, doing what they are "supposed" to do.

It's the same thing that I see with people running on the street, just out going through the motions because that is the way they are "supposed" to lose weight.

What if I told you that that will never work?

Sure, you may hire a trainer, get put on a plan for your exercise and diet, and lose some weight. You'll look awesome, buy new clothes, and probably quit seeing the trainer. You'll stop going to the gym, return to the way you were eating, and find yourself back where you started.

It goes this way with the fad diets people follow as well.

So if you are not having fun with your exercise, why are you doing it? It's just a question to ask yourself, because this all has the potential to be fun! It's just a choice. So why choose something that doesn't get you excited?

Quite simply, if you choose a movement or exercise that you like to do, you will continue with it. It won't be a drudgery to go and do, and *gasp,* you'll lose weight!

So what physical movement really gets you excited?

That one right there!

Go do it!

Or maybe not. Because you really wouldn't want to be happy with the exercise you do!

What patterns of the past are you hanging onto and why?

Are you still eating the same way you always were? Are you still working out the same way as well?

Or maybe you just spend your free time watching TV and complaining that you can't lose weight.

What about your patterns and habits are moving you forward, and which ones are holding you back?

Honestly! It is comfortable in there, in that warm familiar place called your habits.

But you will not get anywhere new from there. Never has happened, never will.

Have you ever heard something like, "Beauty lies beyond your comfort zones"?

Your life exists there too.

Yes, it does.

Your death exists in your cocoon– a slow, boring death.

If you truly wish to create something new with your body, you have to be willing to try something new with it. Consider a new way of eating, for example. I am not suggesting trying new "diets."

God, that word.

But what about gaining awareness about your habits and the effect that they have on your body and your life? What about taking stock of the ones that are working for you and the ones that aren't? It is quite possible that habits which worked in the past are not working now. Does that mean just because they worked before that you should stay with them?

There's that comfort zone again.

What if you stepped out into something new? Almost anything new?

Do you think your body would respond to the change? Would you like to try?

What if you created your life truly moment by moment? What if you stopped using the past as a way of determining what it is you should do now?

Is it at all possible that you are a different person now? Encountering an entirely different set of circumstances? They may look the same, but the game can and has changed.

I know, what do we have if we don't use our wisdom, our experiences to guide us along?

How about using your awareness? Do you know what the difference is? Awareness is that knowledge of what to do before your brain gets in there and distorts it with judgment.

Follow your Bliss!

Yes, this is the name of the book, but for this I would like you to consider the movement you are choosing to do.

Quite simply, do the movements or exercises that make your soul sing, whatever that is.

These are the movements that you will stick with and do on a regular basis without feeling heavy about it.

What does that mean? You will do these movements without hesitation.

I can't tell you how many times I have had clients in the gym because that was where they were "supposed" to be to lose weight and to get into shape. They would force themselves to get there. I began telling people that the best thing I offered as a personal trainer was that I was an accountability partner.

Fine. But what if you didn't need an accountability partner to get through your exercising? What if you didn't have to just get through your exercising? What if it was FUN?

If it was FUN, wouldn't you look forward to doing that?

For many years I worked out in gyms. I looked forward to it. It is fun for me to go in and hit the weights. It is a great way to lose fat and get into shape. For me. Maybe not for you!

So what do you like to do physically?

That! Right there.

The first thought you had.

What if we built your movement plan around that?

The Gym as a Lie

This is one of my favorite places in the entire world!

The gym.

The banging around of the weights, the camaraderie among all of the lifters, the smells of chalk, rubber, even sweat.

When I walk in that door to the Church of Iron, my mind and mood shifts. It's time to get after it. I feel comfortable there. I feel at home. I have seen something in the years that I have been a trainer: I've seen people who are intimidated, unsure of themselves, even scared to be in there. I've had to console, cajole, and push people in the gym. I've had to drive them past their comfort zones to accomplish something they never thought possible. I've had to call or text them to make sure they were coming into the gym for their sessions.

I've gotten pretty good at creating a space in there with a client, a sort of bubble that only the two of us are in.

The focus is just on us and the client's workout. Forget that there are 50 to 100 or more other people in the gym. It has become so popular in modern society to say that the gym, and the workouts provided in them, is the best and sometimes the only way to successfully lose weight and get into shape. People buy this story as their own.

This point of view is where the gym as a lie is created. We get into the idea that it is just necessary to go through the 60 or more minutes, 3 to 5 times a week, even though we really don't like being there, lifting weights, and walking on treadmills. Why?

In the years that I've been a trainer, I've come to the awareness that the gym is not the place for a lot of people.

Yup! I said it! The gym is a lie for a lot of people! It is not their truth. So why continue to go?

The one thing I have figured out about these people is that it's rare to see any significant success from the programs put together for them, whether I am the trainer or not.

The stress of the gym environment, the structure of the workout and eating plans are just too much to overcome. These people are not having fun!

To top it all off, we have the judgments that comes with the industry of personal training, body building, and society – the ones that tell us if we don't do things a certain way, look a certain way, or eat a certain way that we are unworthy.

How is it that we figure we can solve a problem for a person, which was created by judgment, with more judgment?

So what is your truth? What type of movement or exercise totally gets you excited when you think about it? Or at least, what sounds fun?

What if you did that on a regular basis? Would you look forward to doing it on a regular basis? And what kind of change can you create for your body with that?

The Fitness Industry is a Lie!

Yes, it is! For the most part.

It is designed to take your money first and deliver results second. And most of the time, trainers, gyms, and programs believe that they have the only way to lose weight! Just follow their plan exactly, no deviation, and you will lose weight! But what if their plan isn't right for you? What if it is difficult for you to follow? And what if you can't catch on to it?

What happens then? Is it possible that we are creating an environment for failure for most people?

First I'd like to say, what if there is nothing wrong with you? What if you haven't failed at this, but you just found a way that doesn't work for you? And what if that is a triumph?

Stop and think about how many times an inventor found ways to get around the fact that what they were trying to do didn't work. What if he or she had given up at that first "failure"?

What if the fitness industry, or more precisely fitness trainers, took this into account and really worked to find a plan that would work for you, not just try to shoehorn you into a plan that worked for them, or a plan they read from their favorite fitness author?

How does that feel for you to hear?

What Movement or Exercise is Right for You?

There is a lot of information out there about what is the best way to lose weight, get into shape, and to build muscle. So many opinions abound, how can you tell what to do?

And really, what is the right movement or exercise for you? How do you tell?

Well, it is really simple.

Think about that movement, exercise, or game that gets you excited. Maybe it's an activity you used to do when you were younger and stopped because you got a job, a family, or were told by someone that you are an adult now!

Right? How silly is that?

The simple part of this is that the exercise that you like to do, and will do often, is the right one to help you lose weight. If you don't like what you are doing, and you are forcing yourself to do it because you have to, it has very little chance of becoming a lifelong habit!

So think about it. What movement is fun to do?

Do that! Often!

If You Choose the Movement for Yourself, How Does that Feel?

What if no matter what choice you made, you aren't wrong?

Some may benefit you more than others, but the point here is to know that you can choose whatever you like. And know this: If you stop enjoying your choice, choose again. As a matter of fact, you don't have to do the same thing all the time.

What would it feel like to run one day, play with your kids the next, go for a long hike another, swim one day, then ski on the weekend? See where I'm going here? Make it fun. Mix it up if you would like! Just get out and move your body!

How to Create a Movement Plan for Yourself

This seems like a mystery to a lot of people. I know.

Most of the time I get hired because I know how to create a movement plan, and it can be a bit of work to research how to build one that fits the person and keeps it mixed up and interesting.

How can you go about doing this for yourself? I like having clients for what I do in the gym with people. I really enjoy this part of my day! But I also like empowering people to do it themselves. It gives me a great thrill to see clients leave me and continue to work out in the gym, knowing I had a hand in giving them the confidence and the knowledge to do it themselves.

But what about doing it yourself from the beginning, maybe even without the gym?

There are no rules to this—really!

There are, though, a few things that you can do to maximize your time.

Know this first: Just get out and move! It will have an effect on you. Our bodies are built to move. Muscle and bone strength depend on it. Your lymphatic system relies on regular muscle contraction to move those toxins and infections out of your body. Digestion depends on movement.

Constipated a lot? Get out and move. Just move!

Now, if you are looking to maximize your results, let's look at a couple of different things you can do. Make this movement a regular part of your week, day even. Whatever movement that you pick, plan to spend about 60 minutes doing it.

I just heard you: You don't have time to do this.

Now, think about how much time you spend each day watching TV. What if you replaced an hour of TV time with your chosen exercise?

Hmmm....

Now, spend around 10 minutes warming up. This could be stretching, or just an easy pace doing whatever you are choosing to do.

With the main part of your "workout" you could utilize alternating periods of faster then a slower pace. The idea is to raise your heart rate, then let it drop a bit, then raise it again. It's based on a tried-and-true method called high intensity interval training (HIIT). And it works!

It's simple to do, and it's effective. The time intervals aren't as important as doing it. Just don't let your heart rate drop back

all the way to resting during your workout. You can use a heart rate monitor if you like. Find out your resting heart rate (take this when you are just sitting), then use it for reference.

Here is another number to keep in mind: Take 220 and subtract your age. This is a good reference number for your max heart rate. The better shape you are in, the more time you can spend near or at this number. When you are just starting out, if you aren't in great cardiovascular health, or you're at an advanced age, stay well below this number.

Lastly, make sure you discuss any and all of this with your health care provider before starting any exercise plan. Please!

Leave a few minutes at the end of your workout to cool down, and stretch. There are a ton of references to stretching online or in your local the library. And that is pretty much it! Change your interval times around from time to time, play with the periods, and see what is working best for you. Remember: just move!

What can the gym do for you?

Our society has elevated these places as the pinnacle of health and fitness — the place you must go if you want to get into shape.

One thing I have found silly over the years was the number of people (myself included) who will drive to the gym to walk on the treadmill or ride a bike! In the winter month in cold climates, and during inclement weather, I get this. But when it is nice out, get outside for this.

So back to what the gym could do for you.

If this place excites you, or at least if you're comfortable there, it can provide an excellent workout, with variety and plenty of ways to create workouts for any goal and to keep things fresh. Most gyms have trainers you can hire to create plans and keep you accountable. Also, the staff can sometimes show you around. I would recommend hiring a trainer if you want proper guidance on form and building a workout plan to fit you. Regular staff may fall a little short on this understanding.

What Happens When You Move Your Body on a Regular Basis?

As I have said before, our bodies are meant to move. We touched on the benefits to digestion, lymphatic system function, and muscle and bone strength.

By just asking your body to do something that requires a different load on it (walking, bike riding, and lifting weights) your bones and muscles compensate by becoming stronger. What does this mean for the health of your body?

Well, for one thing, just 30 minutes of walking a day is enough to keep osteoporosis from happening. Really! That is one of the things good bone density does for you.

Just imagine what happens when your exercise progresses beyond walking for 30 minutes every day?

By asking your muscles to grow stronger, you will handle everyday tasks much more easily. And if you continue to move and to workout, as you age you will be far less likely to lose muscle.

And regular daily exercise can cure depression. Really! It is one of the best natural anti-depressants out there. It's free, and it has no side effects, unless you would like to consider increased health and vitality, more muscle, less fat, and that awesome endorphin kick provided from your workout a side effect!

How about a little further exploration of some of those potential "side effects"?

1: Exercise controls weight

Regular exercise and movement can prevent weight gain and help you maintain the weight loss you may be experiencing with your exercise program. Moving your body more vigorously and beyond your normal, everyday activity level requires calories.

So instead of just storing those calories (as fat) for use another day, your body will most likely use them for the activity, and for the rebuilding of muscle in the days that follow. If you are having trouble finding time to exercise during the day, start by adding more movement to your day: Use the stairs instead of the elevator or escalator. Park further from the door at work and at stores. Take a walk during your lunch instead of just sitting around after eating.

2: Exercise can keep you healthy and prevent diseases
Regular activity boosts high-density lipoproteins (HDL) or what your doctor calls "good" cholesterol. It also decreases unhealthy triglycerides. What does this do for you? Well, it keeps your blood flowing smoothly, which decreases your chances of cardiovascular diseases like heart disease, high blood pressure, and stroke. Regular physical activity will reduce or manage a host of conditions such as metabolic syndrome, type 2 diabetes, depression, cancer, and arthritis.

3: Exercise can improve your mood
Feel a little low or concerned about something in your life? That exercise you choose to do, whether a workout in the gym, a bike ride, or a walk will elevate the "feel good" chemicals in your brain and give you a much needed boost. You may even start feeling better about your appearance with the continued activity level. Can you use a little more self confidence? I have found nothing else that gives me a better boost in self confidence than the accomplishment of a great workout.

4: Exercise boosts energy
When your body is functioning better, your digestive system is flowing, your lymphatic system is moving toxins out of your muscles and organs, your mood is improved, and your

mental clarity is there. All because of the increased oxygen and nutrients to your tissues, you find more energy to handle your everyday chores.

5: Exercise promotes better sleep

Are you not sleeping well? Try exercising and see if that helps put you to sleep better, deeper, and longer. What would that do for you?

6: Exercise = better sex life

Too tired, or have you lost the desire for physical intimacy? Remember that mention of the boost in self confidence and feeling better about your appearance because of exercise? Do you think that might translate to the bedroom?

Besides, regular exercise can lead to enhanced arousal for women, and reduced chance of erectile dysfunction in men. Sound like more fun?

7: Exercise can be fun (speaking of fun!)

Plan your exercise time with a friend or loved one. It can be a fun, bonding experience! Pick fun activities for the two of you, or the group you are with. I like or bike a trail, join a recreational league, or find a meetup.com group with the same likes as you. And if you get bored with the activity, know this… you can always try something new.

Excess Post Exercise Oxygen Consumption (EPOC)

I thought I would talk a bit about this because it explains why certain types of workouts are more effective than others.

The HIIT type training is one that creates this effect. This is simply the amount of oxygen your body will use after a workout to recover and rebuild. The more oxygen your body requires to recover; the more calories you will burn.

But that isn't a license to overdo it! More is not necessarily better. With a HIIT session that includes resistance training (weights), you can experience this effect for up to 72 hours, burning calories the whole time that you otherwise wouldn't burn them. It becomes a much more effective weight loss workout than just steady state cardiovascular work like walking on a treadmill. With the walk on a treadmill, the preferred workout for those looking to lose weight, your calorie consumption due to the workout ends the minute you step off of the treadmill.

So think about this: you can spend an hour on the treadmill, burning around 500 calories total, or set up a HIIT workout anywhere and continue burning calories for the next couple of days: Which would you choose?

Cardio

The short of this is, if you really like running, walking stairs, or riding a bike or elliptical for hours every week, then go for it! If this is your sole means for exercise, and fat loss is your goal, adding at least a few cycles of HIIT into your workout sessions will benefit you far more that just steady state cardio work.

Workout Anywhere?

We don't need no stinkin' gyms!

Yeah, I am a personal trainer and former body builder and I just said that! You really don't *need* the gym to work out! We've been sold this bag of goods that the gym and the workout possibilities there are THE way to get into shape and lose weight.

In truth, you can work out anywhere! You can turn almost any physical activity into an opportunity to get your body moving and have all the benefits that movement affords you! Yes, the more intense the movement, the more calories you will burn, but it isn't required to completely bust your ass everyday!

Wow! Did I just say that too?

What I am getting at with that last statement is to "program" in some lighter activity days. Your body will thank you for it in ways you can never imagine.

So back to working out anywhere: What movement, sport, activity is it that gives you total bliss? That is what will give you the most benefit. Why? Because that's what you will want to do on a regular basis — so do those!

I know you have been told that the only way to successfully lose weight is to spend mindless time on the cardio equipment in your gym, biking, walking, running your way to optimal health. Guess what? It's not true! It's actually counter-productive for most people.

Unless you are a distance athlete of some sort, or just really dig running, biking or walking fast, there are better ways to lose fat. In fact, the cardio most trainers are prescribing for clients to lose weight becomes a nightmare of quick plateaus, adding more time, more days, on and on until...

Burnout!

Most of the people that I have seen in the gyms doing this kind of workout for fat loss never achieve their goals. They are there the next year, on the same equipment, looking the same or bigger sometimes!

So, now that I've done my part in dispelling that myth, what is it that you would like to do movement wise? Do that!

Metabolic Resistance Training

Metabolic Resistance Training, or MRT for short, is just a fancy way of saying moving fast with weights.

The principle is to combine the benefits of resistance training (weight training) with cardiovascular training. And it is very effective, which is why I wanted to include it here.

You can build an MRT workout just about anywhere, and can do it with just bodyweight for a fairly effective workout. But for those of you that go to the gym, this may be the most effective use of your time there.

It is a simple plan: Combine a string of movements together, one after the other with little or no rest in between. The simplest plan I have found to be effective is like this:

Lower body movement/ upper body movement/ lower body movement/ upper body movement. 4 movements, no rest in between, 10-12 repetitions each.

Your rest happens at the end of the 4 movements. And it's only about a minute of rest—just enough to get your heart rate back down a bit.

Then repeat again as many times as you'd like. Usually if you have set this up well, 5 rounds will be sufficient.

So for a sample workout:

Squats/ pushups/ lunges/ back rows. It really is that simple. Not easy, but simple.

Base your exercise choices on big, multi-joint movements—no arm curls, triceps extensions, or calf raises. Big movements that are more difficult to do will yield results.

The idea here is while your body is recovering from the work of your legs, you do an upper body movement. Then while you are recovering from that upper body movement, you hit your legs again, then back to upper. Then rest everything. This is pretty much the principle behind the Crossfit movement.

Crossfit

This is huge right now, but it will fade away eventually. I know, I hear all of you crossfitters! "This is the perfect workout! It will never fade away!" Yes it will. It will fade away in favor of the next greatest thing. I have one word for you: Jazzercise.

I am not here to pick a fight with anyone on this. Just state a fact. I've been working out or training others for the better part of 30 years now. I've seen things come and go, whether it be the next best workout, diet, etc.

It is the fickle nature of human. We bore easily, and we need to find something new to entertain us. That is all.

Plus the fact that most of the people who pick up a weight will find it difficult, then will continue to move on to something else that promises faster, better losses or gains. We will continue to see the rise and fall of "the next best thing."

I think that Crossfit has succeeded in getting people to work out who otherwise wouldn't. And for that Crossfit has my respect. What I don't like about it is that there is no apparent adjustment for the size and abilities of participants. You do the weight that is prescribed, for as many reps as you can get, competing sometimes against bigger, stronger people. I've been reading about unnecessary injuries doing this workout, so if you choose Crossfit, just beware of your limits. Listen to your body.

Won't weight training make me too big and muscular?

I hear this all the time. Women are afraid that even touching a weight will cause them to gain too much muscle and look like a man. And the men tell me from time to time, "I want to get into shape, but I just don't want to look like you. You are too big!" Cool.

I am here to tell you, it won't happen. Even for men, this is a target that requires a commitment that most won't have. It is a bliss all to itself. And when you have that bliss for the process for building muscle, everything comes simply. Not easily, but simply. And it will feel like the best feeling in the world to you! You can't wait for that next workout!

This is what fuels the process of getting bigger muscles. Everything else in your world just becomes second. This, the sustained, day after day, week after week, month after month, year after year commitment to this process is what builds muscle.

A man would have to desire it like nothing else in this experience! If he doesn't have that kind of desire for building muscle, then he won't achieve it.

And for women, the process is even tougher. Women are not really built to build big muscles. They are hormonally built to bear children — a requirement very different than men. Women will store fat easier, because fat is an amazing source of the calories needed to bare children. Women are not built to build big muscles, because genetically, or at least in the story we have here in this reality, bigger muscles are not required of her to move society along.

Men do the lifting, building and hunting. Thus, there is a need to be muscular. Still though, even for men, building an exaggerated physique is an effort! So if it is something he desires to do, he should get into the gym and lift weights! That will provide just what he requires and no more.

Hiring a Personal Trainer

There are a couple of things I want to share on this topic. The choice of hiring a personal trainer to help guide you to better health and wellness is a big step, one that could potentially ruin the journey before it gets started. Why? Because hiring the wrong trainer for you can make the whole experience of training suck so bad that you will leave the experience with a bad taste in your mouth about trainers– and about the process of training altogether!

Feeling defeated, you may just give up all together, never seeking out another trainer or another way of achieving your target! So, first and foremost, find the trainer that resonates with you. Identify the one who just "feels" like the right trainer.

This will most likely be the one that you will enjoy the most over the course of your working with him or her. A connection with this person beyond just "do this many reps, eat this food' will go much further in your quest for health and wellness or just an amazing naked body!

Credentials really aren't all that important. The more letters behind your trainer's name does not necessarily mean they are a great trainer, just that they are great at studying and taking tests. The absorption of the material and the practice of working with people in the real world are what can make a trainer great. But do ask about a trainer's background. It is important and relevant to your success with this person.

Your trainer, however, ought to have CPR and first-aid training, and he or she must carry liability insurance. A certification from a reputable organization is good, but not the end all, be all. I've seen trainers with an awesome certification who just plain suck at training people!

The more time a trainer has spent in the gym training people usually translates to him or her being a better trainer. There is something that training people, over time in real world settings, just shows a trainer. The experience is more than any program or certification could ever replace.

Ask for references. See what other people have experienced with your potential trainer. And finally, quit making how much a trainer costs the most important criteria. How much is guidance for a healthier, happier you worth? Bargain basement prices, or more? Are you and your body worth $20 an hour? $100 an hour?

Body building and its influence

I can hear you. I don't want to be a body builder! So why are you talking about this?

There is a direct influence that body building has had on the state of training and "getting in shape" in our society! It has been held for some time now, that a body builder's body is the pinnacle of fitness. I am here to tell you now that it is not.

As a former body builder, and one who has been around other body builders for about 2 decades, body building has become an extreme sport.

The effort that goes into becoming a competition-ready body builder is isolating, extreme on the diet, supplementing, and workout front. It often leaves the competitor depleted of water, nutrients, and sleep, which leads into and past the day of competition.

Even though my body looked fantastic the day of my competitions, I can tell you that I was in the worst shape and felt the worst that I have ever felt! And this is the ideal that we have put up and that we use to measure bodies in our society.

Actors train for months and months to get the bodies we see on the screen, only to drop back to an "average" physique afterwards. Our models don't eat to maintain their "sculpted" appearances. This is the effect body building has had on our collective ideal of the "perfect" body.

Bunk!

I have enjoyed the times that I have been "ripped," but maintaining that and keeping some sense of sanity to life is a full-time job!

If that is for you, then by all means go for it! But if you would like to lead a life filled with all that it has to offer, this will be tough.

Body building has also heavily contributed to the way we work out. The proliferation of gyms across this country and the world owe their existence to body building. Let me explain:

There were gyms before, no doubt, but they were the domain of men, mostly. They were dark, dusty rooms filled with iron, sweat, and blood.

Guys got bigger, stronger, and better in there. Then a man showed up on the scene that would change everything: Arnold Schwarzenegger.

Yup! I will give him this credit!

If it hadn't been for him and movies like *Pumping Iron*, *Conan*, *The Terminator*, and *Predator*, then mainstream society would really know nothing of body building and what was possible for our bodies in the gym.[XI]

So we went out in search of gyms to "pump up" in, and finding the aforementioned dark, dusty gyms, a market was born.

Gyms for the rest of us! And they sprouted! All over came these well lit, visually stimulating gyms. And with them, came the equipment to service this new audience. Bright, shiny, clean machines, inspired by another legend, not as well known, by the name of Arthur Jones.[XII]

Yeah, well, he came up with Nautilus. Most of you may not know of him, but he kind of revolutionized things in the industry with his line of equipment, which he sold off and so now in addition to Nautilus, they have Bowflex and Stairmaster, and Hammer Strength originated in the Nautilus Leverage Line). He also created a training protocol that is still heavily in use today called High Intensity Training.

There are so many permutations of this now, it's hard to count! But Crossfit owes its lineage to Arthur Jones.

With these two men (there were others no doubt) we had the recipe for a movement, and a big one at that! The visual exposure (Schwarzenegger) and the equipment and workout protocol (Jones) to fuel an explosion!

We set out to get ourselves fit using gyms, sometimes forgetting there are other ways to get into shape.

So many people descended on these gyms in search of a fitter, trimmer body, each with his or her own reasons and needs.

We had and have eager gym salespeople to put you into a gym membership. Thousands upon thousands of people sign up yearly for this, thinking this is the way that they will finally lose that weight that they have been carrying. Some do. Most, unfortunately, realize that this requires action and patience and then stop going, never to use their memberships again after about a month or two. They leave soured on the whole idea of working out, and of movement in general sometimes!

The gym isn't the holy grail of exercise! For some of you, a lot of you, the gym is the wrong place. It is full of unfamiliar equipment, it's a new noisy environment, and it's sometimes intimidating. It can be full of judgment, from others and from yourself!

It might create a stressful environment that can add to the issue that drove you into the gym in the first place.

Body building definitely raised the awareness of exercise in our society, but by creating an industry that preys on the hopes of the population by creating itself as the go-to way to lose weight, have we done ourselves a disservice? What happens if we explore the exercise and movements that give us joy like I've talked about in previous chapters?

How about fun, joy, bliss, and the possibility that we may stay with those exercises as part of our lifestyle?

Free Weights vs. Machines

I am asked about this one often. Which is better?

They both have their place.

The machines are good if you are looking to isolate a muscle group or just want to get a quick workout in, without the fuss of putting on and taking off the weights. You can usually just put the pin in the stack and go.

Machines can also be a space-saving option if you have limited space like in a house. A lot of companies make a universal type of machine that has a couple of weight stacks and stations on it for a variety of exercises.

Free weights, however cumbersome and space-hogging they may be, offer a better workout. Why? Free weights will always challenge your body more that their machine counterparts.

To lift a dumbbell, barbell, or kettlebell requires stability and balance. Machines, due to the nature of how most of them are created, handle some of that for you. So why would this stability and balance requirement be better? More muscle recruitment, more need for growth, more calories needed to perform the exercise. Also, free weights require your body to work multiple parts in concert with each other, which will provide you with better carry-over to daily life — and to any other game or sport in which you may participate.

This leads us into:

Full Body Workouts vs. Body Part Split Workouts

What is the difference?

Body part split workouts were born in the body building world. They have you focusing on one body part at a time, like a chest workout, back workout, or leg workout. This allows the person working out to focus on that body part and expend his or her energy on just that body part.

It is a great protocol for body building, but not as good for athletes or just the average gym goer looking to maximize his or her time in the gym.

Why? The time commitment can become a bit longer — or at least it's safe to say that the amount of time spent in the gym could be better utilized with a full body workout.

Most of us will never require that jacked, ripped, and well-developed body of a body builder. So what if you took that time in the gym, that hour you set aside 3 to 5 days a week, and worked your whole body each time?

You could structure your workout to utilize the time you would be just resting in between sets to work another body part- one that isn't related to the one you just did.

For example: Do a squat followed by a bench press. Then repeat. Or you could string a few exercises together like so: Squat, bench press, lunge, dumbbell row. Then repeat. You rest period comes at the end of the string of exercises you put together.

Better maximization of your time in the gym, more calories burned, better recruitment of muscles equals better performance transfer to your life. And of course, a trimmer body!

Chapter Four

Putting All of This Into Action

What would a program look like keeping in mind the questions asked here- and all of the questions that will undoubtedly come up? The world of fitness, full of and run by judgment, may not work for you. It may add to the stress that you already feel, making it all but impossible to achieve what it is that you are looking to do.

Food, Nutrition, Meal Planning

The meal plans designed by nutrition and fitness experts can be difficult to follow. There are too many rules, too much structure and denial. These meal plans can be followed, and done well, if a person maintains focus on the end goal. I know this, because I design meal plans from time to time to get myself into shape for a body building contest, or a trip, or just when I feel I have "let things go" for too long. It is difficult to follow these strict meal plans, and I am finding it increasingly difficult as I gain more awareness of life.

A big part of the process I have come to discover is learning to "listen" to your body — listen to what it is trying to tell you about the food it needs for proper functioning. This can be a difficult task, especially with the added task of cutting through the clutter of marketing with which food companies bomb us, daily, as they vie for our dollars. This marketing will stick in our memories and alter the messages we receive from our bodies.

For example, your body may be telling you it needs some fat and salt. When filtered through the marketing lens in our brains, it may mean that our food choice becomes a Big Mac, large fries, and a Coke. That meal would fit the bill for the fat and salt, and much more than that! This isn't a problem once in a great while; it's when people duplicate this meal day after day, and meal after meal, that they create a situation that may or may not really suit them.

I know what you are thinking: I don't eat McDonalds. I know you don't. But we do a lot of similar things. Do you ever eat pizza or pasta from a restaurant? What about sandwiches, cake, ice cream, chips, cookies, juices, and Gatorade? How about that Starbucks drink you have every morning? You get the picture?

The sum total is what is killing us, a little here, a little there, all adding up over time to introduce health issues like diabetes, hypertension, I.B.S., colitis, and Chrons Disease to our lives.

The Plan goes like this:

Eat when your body tells you to eat. But if you get stuck, think in terms of 4 to 5 "meals" per day. This will help maintain energy and boost your body's metabolism, allowing you to burn more calories during the day. I have compiled a list of foods below that come in 4 categories.

Eat anytime foods: These are foods that you can eat anytime you wish, as long as it is feeding a need your body is asking for. It is unlikely you will overeat these. So knock yourself out!

Eat sometimes foods: These are foods (carbohydrates mostly) that can give you issues in terms of weight loss, if they are eaten too often. They are also somewhat addicting and can easily be overeaten. Keep these foods to once per day. No more than two servings a day on the fruit.

Eat seldom foods: As the heading says, these are foods that we should restrict to just once in a while—maybe maybe once or twice per week.

Eat at your own risk: These foods are notorious for causing rapid weight gain and in all honesty are comprised of poisons to our bodies. There are a lot of chemicals used to keep these foods looking and tasting fresh—and helping to keep them cheap! Think of it in terms of alcohol: It's OK once in a while, because your body can deal with the poison. But drinking alcohol everyday to excess can create a problem for you. It's the same with processed and fast foods.

And as I have heard a very wise person say, if you are listening to your body as it tells you what it wants to eat, why would it choose fast food?

A couple of other tips I have learned to consider:

Try keeping your simple carbohydrate (sugar) intake to before mid-day. Something about how our bodies use sugar for energy makes it more likely to get used up during the day. If we take those sugar calories to bed, we are not expending the calories we would during the day, so they tend to be more likely to be stored as fat.

Watch the combinations of fats and carbohydrates, especially the simpler carbohydrates on the sometimes, seldom, and eat at your own risk lists. These together can interfere with how the body stores and uses energy.

These are just a few things to be aware of as you start thinking about what it will take to achieve the body you have always wanted! Combine this plan with some movement in your day (yes, sweating and breathing heavy is a great thing)! Move those muscles around! If you are training with me, you will have a custom plan to follow. If not, get outside and move around! Play games, ride bikes, run, ski, go to the gym, and move some weights around! Aim for at least 30 minutes 4 or 5 times a week.

On to the foods! I will be continuing to update this list as I find more and more to add, or as I shift foods around.

Eat anytime foods:

Proteins
Organic free-range whole eggs and egg whites
Organic grass-fed beef
Organic free-range chicken
Wild game (venison, bison, boar, elk, etc.)
Organic lean cuts of pork
Organic cottage cheese (if dairy is well tolerated)
Whey protein powder

Carbohydrates
Sweet potatoes
Brown rice
Gluten-free oatmeal (100% rolled oats or Irish oats)

Vegetables

ArtichokeLettuce	Onions	Radish
Leek	Spinach	Turnips
Asparagus	Broccoli	Cucumbers
Mushrooms	Peas	Carrot
Kale	Squash	Swiss chard
Beans	Brussels sprouts	Cauliflower
Okra	Peppers	Collard Greens
Shallots	Sweet Corn	Celery
Beets	Cabbage	Tomatoes

Fruit

Blackcurrant	Raspberries	Cherry
Cranberries	Blueberries	Strawberries
Blackberries	Pomegranate	

Fats

Avocado
Raw or dry-roasted nuts (except peanuts)
Natural (100% nuts) nut butters
Olive oil
Coconut oil
Macadamia nut oil
Walnut oil
Grass-fed butter

All spices are allowed and encouraged.

Eat Sometimes foods:

Protein:

Non-organic cuts of:
Beef
Chicken
Turkey
Pork
Organic Greek yogurt (if dairy is well tolerated)
Organic free-range turkey

Carbohydrates

Whole grain breads and cereals (without added sugars)

Fruit

A little word about why I put the bulk of fruit options here: Fruit, even in the conventional training circles, is considered a neutral food, which means that the nutrients (vitamins, minerals, phytochemicals, and fiber) balance out the sugar (mostly fructose) that the fruit contains. This would not have been a concern before we began growing and cultivating fruit for mass consumption. The fruit has been selected for its qualities such as size, flavor, and sugar content to make it the most appealing to the population to buy. Sweeter, tastier fruit means more people buy it, and thus more profit is made. So most of the fruit of today has a much higher sugar content, and yes, nutrient content as well, than fruit of the past.

The other thing to consider relative to the past? Fruit was not readily available, so it was a once in awhile treat Rather than a staple for everyone's diets.

Apple	Pear	Guava
Nectarine	Coconut	Lemons
Apricot	Pineapple	Kiwi
Orange	Fig	Limes
Banana	Plum	Mandarin Orange
Papaya	Grapefruit	Mango
Clementine	Watermelon	Melon
Peach	Grapes	

Eat seldom foods:

Carbohydrates

Crackers
Chips
Cookies
Baked sweets (cinnamon buns, muffins, cupcakes, cakes, etc...)

Eat at your own risk foods:
Most foods from a fast food place
Most frozen dinners

There you go! By sticking to the eat-all-the-time list, you will yield the best fat loss results!

The Lean Tool:

Okay, this is an Access Consciousness tool to help with awareness around food and what your body desires. Hold the food you are considering eating in front of you right about your solar plexus (the area around your diaphragm). Ask your body if it would like this food.

If you lean into it, that would be a yes. If you lean away, that would be a no. If you waver to one side or another or no movement at all, your body may need more information.

There may be an ingredient in there that your body doesn't want. Or it may like to have another item just like it. For example, if you pick up a strawberry and you lean to the side, try another strawberry and see what happens. It may have not wanted the energy or something else inside the one, but the other would work just fine. As with anything else here, keep asking questions!

**Exercises for your beautiful mind,
emotions, thoughts, and spirit:**

I have made workouts available to you for download at:
www.ConsciousGreg.Com/BlissWorkouts

It happens. We find ourselves caught up in the thoughts of what we could've done better in the past, or the worry of what may come in the future. That is fine. It's all part of the experience of life. We are given these abilities as tools to help us, to guide us along.

But what happens when we get lost in that space? Does it remove the bliss in embodiment experience? It sure can!

So what can you do when you find yourself in a loop of one or the other?

First of all, I would encourage you to remember this: The past does not belong to you anymore. Only the memories belong to you. Therefore, there is nothing more you can do about what happened back then. Besides, if you use the tools of the memories, you are no longer that person. So, why dwell there?

The future also does not belong to you. Not yet. Nothing ever really turns out the way our minds create them with our worrying. So why waste your imagination that way?

Also, the future's path is not laid out for you. You get to choose that by your thoughts and actions. How do you do that? Certainly not by keeping your head in the past or in the worry of the future.

You choose your future by being in the present. This is what you have. It is where you get all the awareness of the next right step. The next actionable thought comes when you are in the present.

Could that be why it is called *the Present*? It is a gift.

Now, how do you bring yourself into the present when everything in your mind is going a hundred miles an hour with the thoughts of what happened or what may still come?

Here is a simple exercise that I use to do just that:

(Reference from pg. 11)

> Close your eyes if you like.
>
> Feel your breath.
>
> Inhale and exhale.
>
> Focus on this: In and out. In and out. Over and over.
>
> Feel that? Do you feel your chest and abdomen rising and falling?
>
> Notice how that just pushed everything out of your head? All those thoughts had no room to exist in your consciousness just then.

Now, keep doing it. What else is in your immediate surroundings? Sights, smells, feelings, people?

One reminder exercise that I use all the time now (because it is what caused me to develop this practice in the first place) is spending time with my daughter. Why would I waste any precious moment with her on some thoughts about what already happened, or what may or may not come? My time with her here is finite. She is getting older day by day!

What I found myself doing one day is worrying about money, about how I was going to pay bills, and not paying attention to what I was doing with her. I thought to myself that this will not do! I did this exercise and began to focus only on what is in front of me in that moment.

What I got from this was an enjoyment (read: Bliss in Embodiment) that I wasn't enjoying. And as for those bills? Well, the awareness of how to take care of them came along. Clients showed up for me in times I could never have predicted.

The worry I had for the future was a waste of my time, imagination, and the time and enjoyment for my daughter as well. She now has her Daddy in the present with her much more often.

When I find myself in that space again, drifting to the past or the future to the point that it absorbs my present, I stop and do this exercise to bring me back here. It works every time. You don't have to use my example. You may not have children. How about a spouse, friend, or pet?

How about your job, exercise, hobby, the abundance and beauty of what is around you — the air, rain, snow, sunshine, clouds, moon, stars, trees, grass, or music?

Do you see what I am getting at here? You always have something in your world at the moment that you can connect with to bring you into the present.

Reprogramming your dominant thought patterns

When I realized that I had a dominant thought pattern running in the background so to speak, in my subconscious or even unconscious mind, I saw how that could be running the whole show for me! Whether the dominant thought was one that supported my success as a body builder or any of the endeavors I have taken on, or if it was a thought pattern of failure, it runs the show.

Dr. Wayne Dyer has explained it well, and he has also offered ideas about how to reprogram these patterns.[XIII] So what follows is a bit about what he has said and my interpretation of it, as well as the practice that I use for myself.

Consider the last job you had and consider how you had to spend time and conscious effort learning the new position, step by step. You had to consciously repeat those steps over and over until you had it wired, so to speak. It became second nature, right?

This is the place where you could now do your job and carry on any other task without messing up your job task, right? The processes of your job are now running in the background. Your subconscious is doing it for you.

Think about that when you consider the though patterns that may be running in the back of your mind. These may be thoughts about your worthiness, your beauty, your lovability, or your ability to accomplish something. You may be telling yourself over and over that you are fat, ugly, a dork, whatever. These thoughts run in the background all day long.

So what do you think that they may be doing for you? And how will the universe or your body as well respond to this?

Whether you agree with me or not about how the universe responds to thoughts and feelings is immaterial here. Your thoughts set the mood for you to go about creating your world.

So what would it be like to have thoughts of worthiness there instead, all the time running in the background of your mind? Do you think that would boost your self-confidence? And what do you think you could accomplish with that elevated self-confidence?

So how can you go about reprogramming those thoughts? Think about that job again for a minute…

Think about how you learned those new processes. How you needed to be conscious of them while you were going about the task of learning. You can do this with your thoughts as well. The first step is recognizing the defeating thoughts in your mind. This may be the trickiest step of all, and recognizing when you make defeating or diminishing comments about yourself out loud is a good place to catch yourself and begin the process.

When you hear yourself say something like, "I am fat," or "I suck," or "I can't find someone to love me, take the time to rephrase those statements. Pick anything that stands out positively in your world, in that moment. Just shifting your thoughts to the beautiful weather, your child's laugh, or a smile from a stranger can have an immediate effect on you and your body. You can use this exercise to ease your way into using more positive thoughts about yourself. Those thoughts are there, because there exist amazing and beautiful things about you. By shifting your thoughts just a bit to something positive, you will create space for those thoughts to come through to you.

You will begin to feel the thoughts that are defeating as you go along. They may be different for you than for others, but you will know them.

In the next section I go through a bunch of things that stress out some of my clients, and those stress items can most certainly be shifted with this exercise as well. So when these defeating thoughts pop up, you can begin to reframe them.

Since you have gotten this far in the book, hopefully you have returned to that spot we are born into this world with – that place of being a beautiful, amazing, unique being worthy of all that is good and abundant in this life. So, when one of those negative utterances comes out of your mouth, shift the thought to one that is in support of you being that amazing, beautiful, unique being.

You can also say these statements to yourself throughout the day. When you first get up in the morning, feel that amazingness! Feel your beauty! Feel how magical you are! State it to yourself! State how worthy you are of all the abundance in the universe! State how lovable you are! Do this enough, and the dominant pattern of your thoughts will shift. I promise! What will follow in your life is just amazing!

To follow are a couple of lists that my clients have handed into me. One is a list of common stressors in life; the other list is one of common things that bring joy and bliss. I've added thoughts, questions, and ways that I have gone about dealing with the stresses of life and included ways to boost the things that bring joy.

Stressors

Finances:
This is a common stress to have – probably the most common one. Why is that? It is one that has plagued me throughout

my life. Until I snapped myself out of it. I discussed it at length in the exercise bringing your thoughts and yourself into the moment. This was the best thing I did for myself and my money flow!

What I figured out there was that worrying about money was robbing me of the bliss of the moment, which was also robbing me or the ability to "hear" the awareness of how to bring the money into my world to pay bills. So not only do I miss the bliss of the moment when I worry about money, I also miss the opportunities to make the money as well.

I am not suggesting here that you don't take steps to plan your financial future, just that the worrying about it is creating a stress in your world and in your body, and it can be a detriment to your health and your Bliss in Embodiment.

Bills:

So what if this is just part of the guide to your journey through life? What if it's a gift to have bills, since it means that you have attracted some comfort or Bliss by creating things into your life?

Weight:

What is it that you are really worrying about when it comes to your weight? Is it your health and the impact that carrying extra fat has on that, or is it some sense that you are not beautiful if you don't look like the models and actors you see on TV or in magazines?

If it is the former that's fine, but do you need to worry about it? And what is that worry doing for you? Does it tell your body to change? Does it change your habits including your thoughts? And will the worry change the possibility of a health concern? Action is what will do these things for you—a shift in the habits surrounding your lifestyle. Your thoughts, your habits about food, exercise, movement, sleep, and stress reduction/ elimination.

If you stress about your weight because you don't look like the models, actors, or even the fitness bunnies in your gym, well, what if you let that one go? If I told you that you aren't going to look like them, how does that make you feel?

Well, hear me out.

Just as I said before, you are a beautiful, amazing, unique being!

But the thing about the images you see in the media is this… they are fake. Yes, every one of them! What we have by the point of consumption (ready for the public to see) is an image of a person who has probably spent months getting ready for that moment — training and manipulating diet, tanning, taking drugs, applying cosmetics, choosing the right clothes and lighting, where the camera filters and angles.

Then we get to the photo-shopping of the image, which never looks like the person who was photographed in the first place!

As far as the actors in a movie role? They have trained and dieted nonstop leading up to the movie, usually with trainers, chefs, and handlers taking care of all of the process along the way. It is their job to get into that shape! And once the movie is shot, it's off to the next role and preparation for that one.

The fitness bunnies and body builders in your gym are the same. It is a moment in time for them. I know, because I have lived it a few times now in my life. It is difficult to achieve, almost impossible to maintain, and usually unhealthy to get there. Besides, no matter what you choose to do in your life with your body, you will always be the best you that you can be, at that moment in your life!

If you are worrying over someone loving you only if you look a certain way, ask yourself something: Is that person worth your love and affection?

Unconditional love is just that. Unconditional! Having to look a certain way to have someone love you is a condition.

Is it possible that that is the stress you are really feeling? Knowing that that person doesn't really love you?

Worrying about diet:

We have made this word into a negative in most people's world. It brings up connotations of deprivation, starvation, eating cardboard, or other things that taste awful.

Do they ever work? There are literally hundreds and hundreds of diets out there all claiming to work. And yes, they can work provided a couple of things are in place: You stay with it; it is the right diet for you to be on (and you only know that if and when you try them, or better yet, when you work with a nutritionist to find the best possibility for you); and, you are ready to do the diet, meaning your thoughts and your lifestyle will support the changes that can happen.

Having said that, these diets will all work for a limited amount of time. Once you body adapts to the plan, progress can slow or stop, hence the idea of working with a nutritionist on this one.

Here is what I don't like about "diets": They never work long term, for all sorts of reasons.

The biggest reason is that for the most part a "diet" is difficult to impossible to stay on forever. Life happens! Temptations to pull you off of your chosen diet are everywhere. To suggest that any one of us can resist that temptation forever and live any semblance of a fun, blissful life is rare.

So what do I suggest?

Work with a nutrition professional that can help you create a lifestyle around food that can sustain you for the rest of your life. Or create one yourself by reading the amazing amount of information provided for free online or in periodicals all over the place. If the content repeats the word "diet" though, consider skipping it.

As far as the worry about dieting? If you take into consideration what I discussed here, it will reduce your stress about it.

Also, what is worrying about your diet doing for you? Is it providing the energy, space, thoughts, and feelings to provide the success you are looking for with it? The energy of worry could be contributing to the situation you are dieting to get rid of!

Learn a few things about what food is, what it is not, what it is doing for you. And the simple guide I have provided for you here in the appendix of this book will give you a great place to start.

Kids:

It's funny, because when I think about this one, I think about the fact that we were all kids once, with parents and guardians that looked after us and probably worried about us as well!

How did we turn out? How did you turn out? Are you in one piece, a loving, caring, contributing member of a family and society? What do you think you are showing your children by being just that?

Most likely your children will be doing similar things to what you did, making some mistakes along the way (it is how we learn the best, by the way), and having triumphs, heartaches, and so forth. By all odds, they will turn out just fine, like you did.

Does the worry protect them? Or does using that energy to show them how to make choices that will support them and their endeavors prove a better use of your time and imagination?

Husband/Spouse Relationship:

My relationship to my 2 now ex-wives did provide me a great deal of stress, until I figured something out that helps me now. Unfortunately, I learned it too late to save my second marriage, but it is helping a great deal with our partnership in regards to raising our wonderful daughter.

It is simple, really– so simple it makes me laugh when I think that I ever chose to live any way differently. *Never change yourself to fit what you think someone else what like you to be, just to be with them, or get them to fall in love with you. And once you are in a relationship, hold that same integrity to yourself. Never change who you are just to try to please your spouse. It will never work.*

Be who you be– authentically you. Allow others to be who they be, and trust that you and they will operate from this place in everything.

Until it changes.

Then you can renegotiate, decide the change is okay with you, or move on. You always have choice.

But being something you are not is like cutting off parts of you to fit into someone's life, having them become interested in you only to find out down the road, as your traits and behaviors return (and they always will) that they don't really care for the real you.

Can you imagine the stress that will provide?

Extended family:

Whatever it is that your extended family is doing to stress you out can always be let go of. It is just a choice you have to make to be vested in the outcome of something with an extended family member, or not. Choosing to not be vested in something does not mean you don't care; it's just the opposite. You do care, it's just that however it may unfold, you will not allow that to sway who you are, or how you will respond to the family member or the event. This can be the same with friends, coworkers, and random people in your day.

Family:

This is an easy stress to fall into. These people are in your day-to-day life, and they have become significant due to the nature of the birth or marriage connection. Is it possible to allow the people in your family to do their "thing" without your vested interest in that? What would it take to care for your family, their lives and interests, but not take on the responsibility of it?

As a matter of fact, this approach could go for everyone in your life, huh?

To do lists:

My father told me something when I bought my first house. He said that homeownership is a job where there is always something to do, fix, buy, build, clean.

There is always a "to do" list involved. You will never be "done." This is part of the journey.

What would it take to see your "to do" list more as the guide to your life — as the fulfillment of the steps to carry you along the way of your path?

Rushing/being late:

I've merged these two because they feel like they go together.

I've caught myself feeling these often. Do these feelings belong to you, or someone else? Maybe they belong to society in general.

I know, it is considered a sign of disrespect to be late, but is all of the stress we put ourselves through before, during, and after worth the outcome?

Has any situation to which you've been late not worked itself out? Doesn't a simple apology usually solve things when is appropriate? No explanation or excuse to diminish the apology, just the apology. And when you are late for some other event, don't things usually work out?

Illnesses:

Is the illness caused by your stress?

I've noticed that my stress level has a direct impact on my overall health. The stresses that you put on your body can lower your immune system, putting you at risk for illness.

I can look back at my second marriage and see the stress I was under as I tried to fit into a mold that my ex -ife was trying to put me into. I never quite fit exactly, which caused the strife between us. I was in allowance for this, so I am not suggesting blame here at all, just that I now can recognize the stress that put on me.

I have never been sick as often as I was in the years I was married to her. Was the stress of trying to be someone I wasn't, and never quite getting there, plus the other stresses of life I've mentioned above too much for my immune system?

The overall lowering of your stress levels will be an amazing gift to your body. It's the ability to handle the viruses, bacteria, and fungi that bombard us on a daily basis that gives us more Bliss in Embodiment.

Cars:

We could just think about all of the things in our lives — houses, cars, boats, TV's, and furniture. They are transients in our lives. That tends to be their nature, designed probably by us to come and go, allowing for more experiences along the way.

Interesting thought here: What if this way of thinking is what is driving the marketplace today? What if it's a programmed obsolescence in the technology, cars, and clothes? Or what if it's the marketing of products that suggests to us that we aren't worthy if we don't have the latest, greatest?

What if you didn't have a vested interest in the length of time something is in your life? What if you instead felt the gratitude for it being there no matter how long?

Wow– there's that gratitude thing again!

Kid's schooling:

This, like everything in our lives, always works out.

My ex-wife and I recently went through this with our daughter. The school in which she is enrolled is coming to an end. It only takes students through kindergarten, and we needed to find where she would go next. The process was one of finding the possibilities for schools, talking to them, finding out about availability and qualifications. Stress-inducing stuff? Yes. It's definitely possible to get stressed about it.

We narrowed it down to the school we wanted to get her into. Even though we explored the idea before the school even opened, there was a waitlist and a lottery to get into it!

Stress? Yes, definitely a possibility!

How did I handle it? I knew that no matter what, this would work itself out. We had done everything we could do; it was now in the hands of others to take our guidance in this issue.

I just didn't stress about it. And what happened? Our daughter got selected in the lottery and was accepted to the school!

Some might think this to be a coincidence. I prefer to think that by me "seeing" the outcome happening is what brought it about.

Meeting people:

Remember this when you are facing meeting people for the first time: People rarely think of you the way you think that they are. Usually no opinions are even formed yet.

Regardless, why would you concern yourself with someone else's opinion of you?

Go into the situation being who you be. The people who are attracted to that energy will show up and they will be a wonderful contribution to your life.

Social situations:

This is kind of the same as above, if what is stressful about social situations is dealing with the new people you may meet.

There is the added stress potential of what you may be responsible for in this social situation.

Try this next time: What if you didn't promise more help than you could reasonably doodle out? Would you enjoy the time there more?

Conflict:

I know this one well. It has been my M.O. most of my life. I just would shrink in the face of conflict, and of course then feel the impact of not getting in and voicing my thoughts about something. I wouldn't stick up for myself, or I would apologize, ask for forgiveness, whatever.

It always seemed to come back to me with much more energy than if I had just put myself in there in the first place.

Once I started facing these potential conflicts more often, I found something interesting:

They usually weren't the conflicts I was expecting — or at least an issue could get resolved much more quickly than if I avoided it all together.

Guess what that brought me?

Yup! More bliss!!

Saying no:

This one is powerful and it's one of the greatest gifts I have given myself: The ability to say no.

It is freedom. It is grace. It allows you to meet people and situations right where you truly are capable of meeting them. The other side of this is that others now get to make their choices based upon your truth.

There is this old adage of "give until it hurts," and that if you don't, somehow you are less than everyone else.

What if you didn't buy into that story? What if you gave what you are capable of giving?

I'll tell you what has happened for me since I've begun saying no: Yeah. More bliss — for me and the others around me as well.

Friendship:

Here you may face the maintenance required for continuing a friendship. My interesting point of view here is that if the friendship has requirements or expectations that go along with it, then it doesn't fall into the realm of unconditional love. Friendships based upon expectation are never long for this world. Treat them as such. No amount of worry or stress will ever change that.

However, the friendships that last take you as you be no matter what, and they move, adjust, and grow right along with you. Now that is bliss in relationship!

These are the friendships worth the nurturing, and it won't feel like a requirement. You won't sense a need to worry over it; it will simply be blissful to engage in.

Feeling helpless:

Feeling helpless is a choice that we make ourselves. It is a state of victimhood we enter in when we drift from our knowing, when we try to "figure out" everything.

We are woefully inadequate at "figuring things out" when we go at it alone. When we go at it without our awareness, our ability to hear what the universe is offering up as possibilities pretty much disappears. When we step away from our knowing and go it alone, there is only so far we can go and only so much we can know, be, and perceive. This creates limitations on what can and usually what does happen. So if you are looking in the direction you think something may happen (for example, money is tight and your bills are pressing), you think that you've got to figure out how to make more money. So you look at the possibilities with which you are familiar.

Well, these are based upon your past and on what worked then. This represents only a very small sampling of the possibilities for you.

When these times in your life show up, and you react in this manner, your world gets shut down into a tight little ball, causing this hopeless feeling. Right?

Well, what if there was another way? This is a way that seems counter intuitive, but it works. Let go.

Let go of the need to figure out. Focus on what is right in front of you.

Try the "bringing your thoughts and yourself into the moment" exercise cited in the Appendix of this book. It will shift your view, open you up to all the possibilities again, and bring you opportunities you won't be able to think of yourself. It may help you be more able to see if your focus is narrowed by the stress brought on by whatever the situation is.

"This too soon shall pass."

Things that bring Joy and Bliss:

I love these, so I have included them to remind you of the possibilities for joy in your life all around you. Keep looking and experiencing them! Put them regularly into your days and watch the things that stress you out disappear.

Cuddles

Beaches

Hugs

The Ocean

Husband

Softball

Being silly with husband

Feeling Helpful

Sex

Dressing up and wearing Heals

Helping Others

Kids (mine and others)

Exercising - lifting weights

Music

Movies

Dancing

Fresh air

Organizing

Traveling

Chapter Five

BE THE CHANGE

"Be the change you wish to see in the world."

Mahatma Gandhi[XIV]

Regarding Bliss in Embodiment, the thoughts that follow were some of the first things that I practiced before I even knew of the idea of Bliss in Embodiment, or about the quote from Gandhi.

His quote has been in my mind every day for the last couple of years. Of course, I had heard it long before that, but it became a guiding force for me a couple of years ago. As I began to step into sharing my thoughts and awareness on consciousness, waking up myself, and sharing with others, I have rolled Gandhi's phrase around in my head.

I have found many different thoughts and awareness's with this, as I'm sure Gandhi did as well. It is my awareness that he felt the space in the statement, and that he intended it to spark a wide variety of thought to begin with.

I thought I would share my awareness and experiences with the quote. These different ways that I have found to express, live, and create my world stem from this simple statement.

The biggest response I get when I mention this statement to my clients and friends is first kind of a blank stare, the kind of look you give someone when you know what was just said was of a profound, life-changing nature, but it flew right over your head. No worries. It got in there.

The next response I get really has to do with protecting oneself. It is one of, "I do want to be that change," or "I will be that change, but only if others start." Others need to change first, and then, and only then, will I change or be the change I wish to see in the world. You will probably be waiting a long while for that, and your sense of peace won't be obtained by waiting for someone else to change first.

How this statement may begin to work for you is entirely unique. And my experience with it is by no means and absolute. It's just my story, my experience– a guide track, if you will. I will ask you to consider possibilities here you may never have thought of, or thought were impossible given your or the world's circumstances. I may ask you to consider changes in your lifestyle that could afford you some more peace and space to create with this statement, just in the form of considerations and awareness.

Shall we get on with it?

Be the change you wish to see in the world

It has become a cliché, an off-the-cuff remark used sometimes to elevate the user above that of the audience it is directed at. Please know, this is not my intention here, but I have seen it used this way. It has become kind of a throwaway comment and I believe the spirit of the statement got lost.

You see, the beauty of this statement is that everything, absolutely everything, begins in the self. All of the events and experiences, whether considered good or bad, are all there in front of you, directed that way by the movie director in your head.

Yup.

It all is there playing out for you.

What you are most interested in for your life, you direct by the thoughts you have. These thoughts are energy, and they work kind of like picking up the phone to call someone. What is on the other end of the line is a matching energy — an energy that shows up for you in your life, right in front of you to be experienced. The next part of this is where you are placing your awareness- or, more like where are you being in your awareness?

Your awareness is infinite.

It is all around.

Omnipotent.

Where are you placing yourself in your awareness?

What are you noticing around you in the life unfolding in front of you? What of the people that show up, the reactions, responses, and behaviors that you get from them?

What is showing up for you on the TV, in newspapers, magazines, social media, and on the internet?

What are you looking to find there?

Is it most likely things to support your prevailing thoughts?

The world is falling apart, this country is in deep trouble, and there are bad people in the world trying to take away your way of life? Does it surprise you when you find evidence of this?

I am not surprised. I find that what I am looking for is right there to be found. I also have found that I can manipulate the events that play out in front of me by how I choose to think.

Why do I believe this way?

The universal principal of reciprocity

The universe knows nothing of right and wrong, good or bad. It only knows of balance. This isn't a balance like we know of, or can imagine; it is a balance of energy. This can only look like the universe knows it can be.

This universal balancing act is beyond the comprehension of our human minds. Sometimes the balance may appear to us in the form of an unjust act of God. But that is the view through a judgmental lens– one that we as humans possess. It is a limiter for us.

Interestingly enough, we can tap into this knowing. It is awareness, and it is free for us to hear and know. We just choose to view it through the same judgmental lens that we may view the reciprocal actions of the universe. If we can hear the awareness and act upon it either by a knowing or by a choice of action before our brains get hold of the awareness and attempt to make sense of it, we can be the knowing of the universe.

Every relationship is reciprocal. When you touch something, it touches you back. We have this amazing capacity to create anything we desire here, through this principle of reciprocity. The key resides in how it is that we feel about ourselves.

Unconditional love is a language that the universe speaks. It is the language that provides everything here. Because this is the language of the universe, and how it operates, reciprocity happens. So whatever it is that we ask for through our thoughts or through our feelings about ourselves, this is what the universe provides proof for in the possibilities that show up for us to choose from.

These possibilities reflect the energy of our thoughts back to us, giving us the path that lies in front. We create this path by the action of our choices, or non choices. The more we create, the more the thoughts we have grow, the more the universe provides possibilities, the more we act upon and choose-- and the cycle perpetuates.

This is the process behind create or die.

Keep creating, and more possibilities show up to propel you forward on your path.

Stop creating, and the possibilities show up to support the life of non creation. This stagnation is not living; it is creating possibilities that do not serve the higher you — what you are uniquely here to express and share.

Doesn't that just feel like a long death instead of living?

Just sayin'!

We can also be creating a life and path that does not serve our higher self- the self that we desire to be, the self that makes our hearts race with excitement. So what happens when you entertain questions about how to bring about and act upon the awareness that comes from being in the space of what you desire? You have no idea how extraordinary you are. If you can embrace that, there is no end to what you can create for your life.

This principle works as a group, society, and humanity as a whole. The predominant thoughts of a people then in turn lights up the possibilities to match that energy. Then we as a people, or our elected officials, monarchs, and dictators pick a plan of action based upon these possibilities.

Know this: These are the only possibilities we see, but not the only possibilities available. You see, there are infinite possibilities. To be able to awaken to this fact and then know that what we are seeing in front of us is merely that which is enlightened by the reflection of our thoughts marks the moment we reach freedom.

Every day, every moment we are putting something into the universe- some thought, some deed, a vibratory pattern that we resonate at in that moment causes the universe to seek balance or equilibrium. It will return that energy to you, to balance what you contributed.

With this idea in mind, how could you use it to create the change you wish to <u>*see*</u> in the world? How would you shift your thoughts to create what you would like to experience?

This is one of the ways we can begin to shift our attention, our awareness. You can start to see something different unfold in front of you. So, what do you wish to see in the world? What would you do to see that? Are there some things you can do to become that?

The answer is yes. But it's entirely up to you.

You must choose.

And the change really will happen at the speed of choice. When you are ready, you will see the world change in front of you.

How about some things I have done to have this happen for me? The first came well before I knew about the statement from Gandhi.

> *I stopped watching the news, reading newspapers, visiting news sites on the internet*

I can tell you with great assurance, the "news" we see and read about in the media is sensationalized, and it's agenda and advertising-driven.

Having worked in media (radio and cable TV) for 13 years, this is what I found: The doom and gloom stories rule the media world, either because of the sort of morbid tongue- in-cheek saying, "If it bleeds, it leads," or because someone has an agenda to push that the story.

That is it. That is what is driving the "news" that we see.

For the most part, these stories are nowhere near as big as they are made out to be in the news. A little nugget of a story can be blown so far out of proportion that you will think the end of the world is eminent.

Remember Chicken Little?

Case in point: In late 2014, the big story became the Ebola virus arriving in America. At the time I am writing this, 2 cases have been confirmed, and you would think that the whole of America was in danger of coming down with this disease — that is, if you watched the news or read the newspaper every day.

The virus is not that easy to catch: You must have direct contact with bodily fluids from someone infected. Nevertheless, the world was ending.

You can look at the news media as well and see agenda-driven stories based on network biases. Whether liberal or conservative, the stories on those news networks are neither fair nor non-biased, or for the most part, far from what is happening.

What we see in those news reports are just the news that is fit to report, or to support a political or fanatical agenda. So why would you want to create your world from that "awareness"? So what would happen if you stopped watching the news, news-based programs, reading the newspaper, and surfing the internet for news?

You may ask, "How will I know what is going on in the world if you don't do this?"

I can tell you now, after 20 some years of not watching the news or reading newspapers, that the "important" stories find their way to me.

Always.

What has this created for me? Peace. Quite a bit more of it then I had when I did engage in the news media. What else is possible now? Well, I have more time to do other things, like creating my life instead of having it come to me in fragmented, slanted pieces.

What would you do with the time you gained back if you didn't watch the news or read the newspapers? This leads me into a newer practice of mine.

Limiting my engagement in conversations about political/social matters

Notice I said limiting. I haven't quit; it's just that I choose a better jumping in place for me. And Part Tow of this is that I rarely, if ever, argue for or against a point of view.

I have a disappearing need to be right.

Everyone has a point of view, and mine is no better or worse– just different based upon my experience in this reality.

So why would I need to argue mine? If mine works for me, do I need validation for it? Do I need to feel superior by being "right"? Would you rather be right, or happy?

This practice is a new one for me, and still requires some level of a conscious effort to follow it. One tool that I use when I find myself caught in the loop of an argument about something that is really taking away from the bliss of my life is this: I state this to myself, or if I feel it is appropriate, out loud: "You are right, I am wrong."

I may repeat it a few times until I pop myself, or the conversation, onto a new track. It works quite effectively.

Be careful using it out loud. You can inflame a conversation really quickly, as it may be considered a condescending remark.

Meditation

We have all heard about the power of meditation, probably over and over from TV shows, the self-help gurus, to that crazy aunt you have to see at holidays.

Traditional meditation is something I do once in a while, and find a lot of help from it when I do. It just works.

What I would like to show you, though, are some alternate ideas that aren't typically considered "meditation," which I do often use. I assure you, they work.

Kinetic meditation

I first heard the phrase "kinetic meditation" used to describe meditative movement from my friend and play-pal Kathy Basel. She is a fantastic thinker, holistic health practitioner, tri-athlete, mountain biker, and skier– and she's an all-around beautiful person. She just got it and nailed it with the phrase.

What I realized in the moment she uttered the phrase was this has been the predominant form of meditation I have practiced my whole life. And it works. I have several ways that I engage in kinetic meditation.

Playing music

Being a drummer is a physical experience. And I can find myself quite lost in the moment of creating music when I play. It is an amazing release of tension and a chance to create moments like none other.

You don't have to be a musician to experience this, though.

Do you still sing? In the shower, car, or karaoke? Maybe you sing with friends, or along with musicians at a show?

Go for it! The release and creation is fantastic! And I've found the same sense in creating music in my studio. Just writing music is a great meditation. You can get this same sense with any artistic endeavor. It is a connection to the universe, to God, or Source. A reaffirmation of where you come from.

Physical Activity:

I workout and lift weights, mountain bike, backpack in the mountains, and go on walks with my girlfriend and her dog. I used to climb rock, ski, and skateboard. I also play with my child in the park or at home. My point here is that there are many ways to experience physical play. Explore them! Explore as many as you desire! There is something quite therapeutic and releasing about physical activity.

A couple of things here: You will find yourself with less time to devote to watching the TV or reading the newspapers. There will be less time spent with any of the hyped up "news" about the world coming in, and less chances for you to adopt points of view about things that are not yours. You get to create your own world, your own reality! How's that for being the change?

Putting it into play and creating your world

This is by no means an exhaustive list of possibilities, just a few that work for me, providing me more peace and bliss in my life, which are the changes I wish to see in the world.

What shows up in your world is entirely your choice. We create everything from the energy of our thoughts. What predominantly circulates in our mind is what will draw energy to you. If you focus on all of the "negativity" going on in the world, that is the energy and reality you will draw to you. If you choose instead to see and be the energy of "positive," your world will change around you.

Not only does this change your experience, but due to the connectivity of everyone and everything, others will feel the effect, simply in how you vibrate (thoughts and energy), in how you show up in their world (you can be a more positive space for them, creating that possibility for them to join you), and hey, by just you being an all-around fun and uplifting person to be around!

You don't need to add or shift this into your life all at once. Try one on for size for a bit and see if anything changes for you in your life.

This is hardly an exhaustive guide about how to have Bliss in Embodiment. I am just offering ideas that I have come to at this point in my life, right here, right now.

Everything that we take into our bodies either by breathing, putting in our mouths, taking in intravenously or through our skin can and do exert their influence upon our Bliss in Embodiment. How much influence—or how much we suffer or enjoy that influence—is entirely up to us.

The pains and enjoyments in our lives are inevitable. How much we choose to suffer or continue to enjoy these parts of our lives boils down to simple choice. Hopefully this book gave you the insight and courage to continue asking questions and to continue seeking awareness about anything in your life.

Greg

Follow your Bliss - Greg Dyer

NOTES

I   I am not entirely sure I have words to describe what Access Consciousness and these two men; Gary Douglas and Dain Heer have meant to my overall development into thinking this way. Much gratitude for them being who they be! See http://www.accessconsciousness.com/.

II   Sometimes no amount of words will do a subject justice. Abraham is a name. A symbol, a feeling. It's evocative yet simple — just like we want our names to be. But who, or what, is/are, Abraham, really? One workshop attendee said, "... *you're a very attractive woman, too.*"Abraham replied, *"We're usually a nebulous mist, so that is quite a compliment." (Laughter)* Louise Hay calls them "some of the best teachers on the planet today." To Dr. Wayne Dyer they are "the great Masters of the Universe!" This is definitely worth checking out. See http://www.abraham-hicks.com/lawofattractionsource/index.php.

III   Max Planck was a 19th-20th-century German theoretical physicist who originated quantum theory, which won him the Nobel Prize in Physics in 1918.

IV   For more information on the Chakras in Indian thought, see http://www.mindbodygreen.com/0-91/The-7-Chakras-for-Beginners.html.

V   Jon Gabriel: Inspirational and amazing transformation that he is bringing to the planet! See http://www.thegabrielmethod.com/

VI   "No One is to Blame" is a song by British musician Howard Jones. The song, in its original version, can be found on his second studio album, *Dream into Action*, which was released in 1985. See https://en.wikipedia.org/wiki/No_One_Is_to_Blame.

VII   See http://www.abraham-hicks.com/lawofattractionsource/index.php.

VIII   85% of the population being inflamed by these foods is sourced from Lyn Genet's book, *The Plan*

IX   Lyn Genet's *The Plan* is a unique look at food and its effect on the body. See http://www.lyngenet.com/.

X   Well, he was Carl Jung! Often referred to as C. G. Jung, was a 20th-century Swiss psychiatrist and psychotherapist who founded analytical psychology. His work has been influential not only in psychiatry but also in philosophy, anthropology, archaeology, literature, and religious studies. He was a prolific writer, though many of his works were not published until after his death.

XI   Aaanoold! See http://www.schwarzenegger.com/.

XII   Arthur Jones founded Nautilus, Inc. and MedX, Inc. He invented exercise machines like the Nautilus pullover, which was first sold in 1970. He was born in Arkansas and grew up in Seminole, Oklahoma.

XIII   WAYNE W. DYER was an internationally renowned author and speaker in the fields of self-development and spiritual growth. Over the four decades of his career, he wrote more than 40 books, including 21 *New York Times* bestsellers. He created many audio and video programs, and appeared on thousands of television and radio shows. http://www.drwaynedyer.com/

XIV   Mahatma Gandhi was the preeminent leader of the Indian independence movement in British-ruled India. Employing nonviolent civil disobedience, Gandhi led India to independence and inspired movements for civil rights and freedom across the world. The honorific Mahatma (Sanskrit: "high-souled", "venerable") — applied to him first in 1914 in South Africa, — is now used worldwide. He is also called Bapu (Gujarati: endearment for "father", "papa") in India.

About The Author

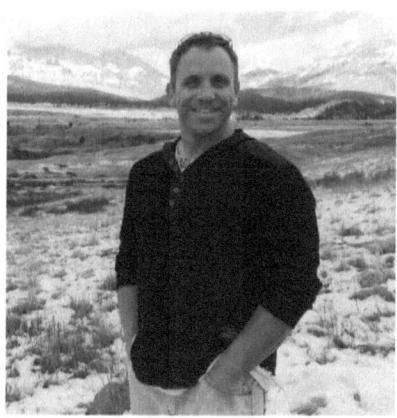

Greg Dyer is an author, speaker, podcaster, mindset coach and trainer.

Greg first found his way into a gym as a shy 16 year old, quickly seeing the physical confidence that came with building his body. This transferred into other areas of his life, including rock climbing and playing the drums. Fascinated by the ability to work with our bodies to achieve anything we thought to be possible, he began studying insatiably things like anatomy, biomechanics, nutrition and exercise programming.

In 2000 he competed in his first bodybuilding competition.

In 2004 Greg became a certified personal trainer to share with others his expertise and love for the human body's capacity. Through the course of training hundreds of clients, one thing came clear to him; the fitness industry model was flawed. Greatly!

What he saw is that the industry has been trying to solve the same problems (things like weight loss and body image) with the same level of judgment that create the problem in the first place!

This led to an epiphany for him. What is the one component that we don't facilitate often in the fitness industry? Mindset.

Not only for being able to visualize yourself being where you desire to be with your body, but all of the thoughts that led to the struggle with body in the first place -- the judgments, expectations, and victimhood that go along with not being authentic in who you truly came to be.

Greg's enthusiasm, passion and experience now all play a part in his refreshing approach to helping his clients master their mindset as the key to achieving the body and the life they desire.

Greg loves being a Father to a beautiful Daughter and continues to enjoy music and outdoor adventures mountain biking with friends all over Colorado and Utah.

"I absolutely love seeing the freedom people enjoy when they achieve something they never thought possible!"

www.ingramcontent.com/pod-product-compliance
Lightning Source LLC
Chambersburg PA
CBHW030444290526
45786CB00001B/441